SKIN

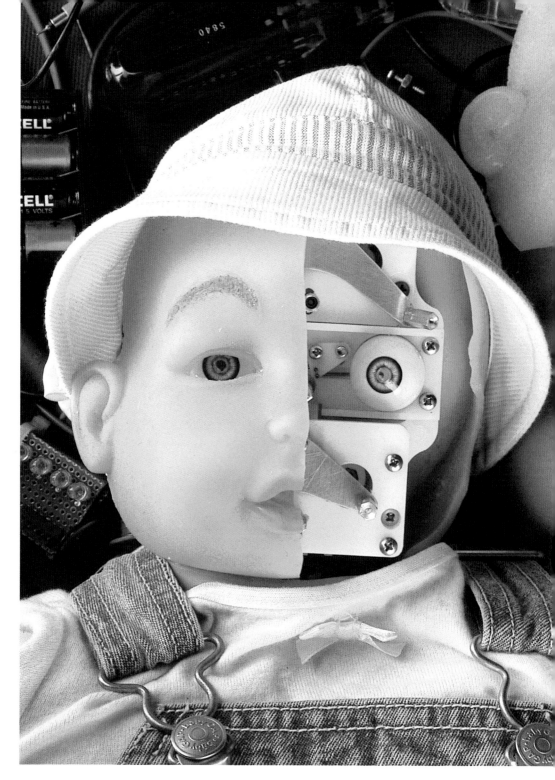

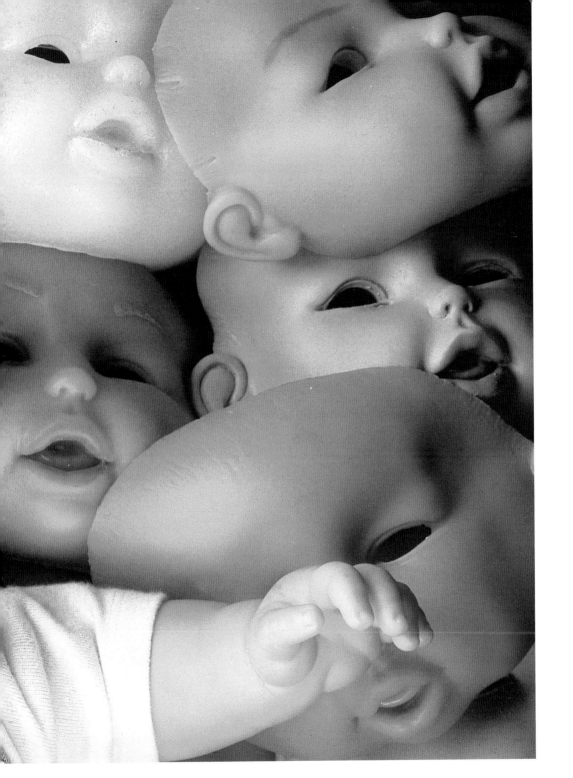

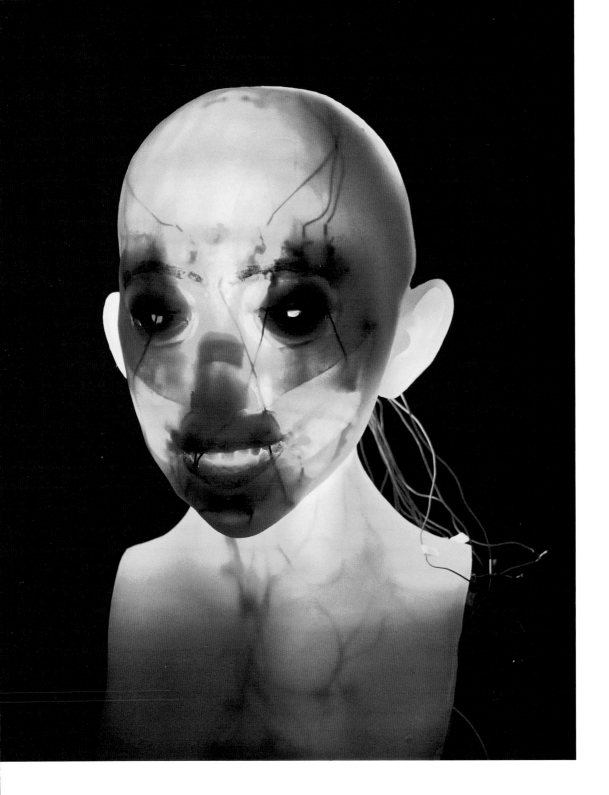

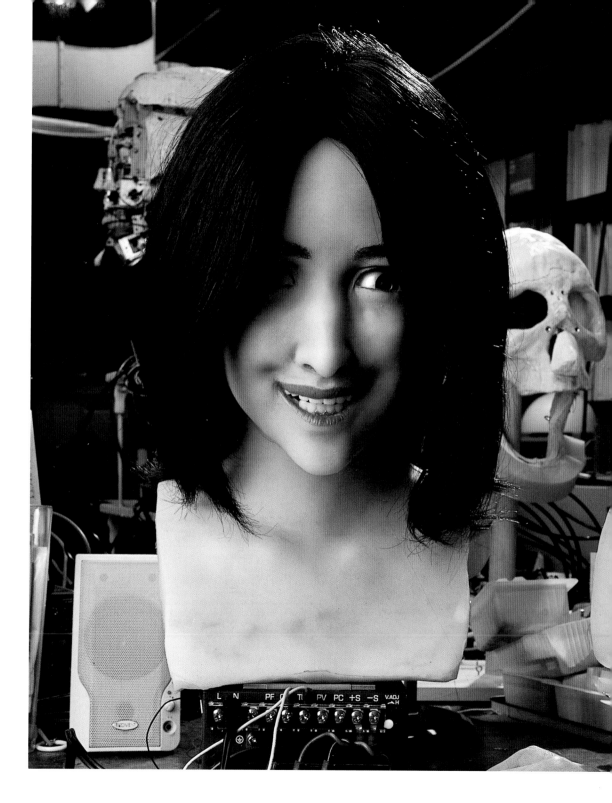

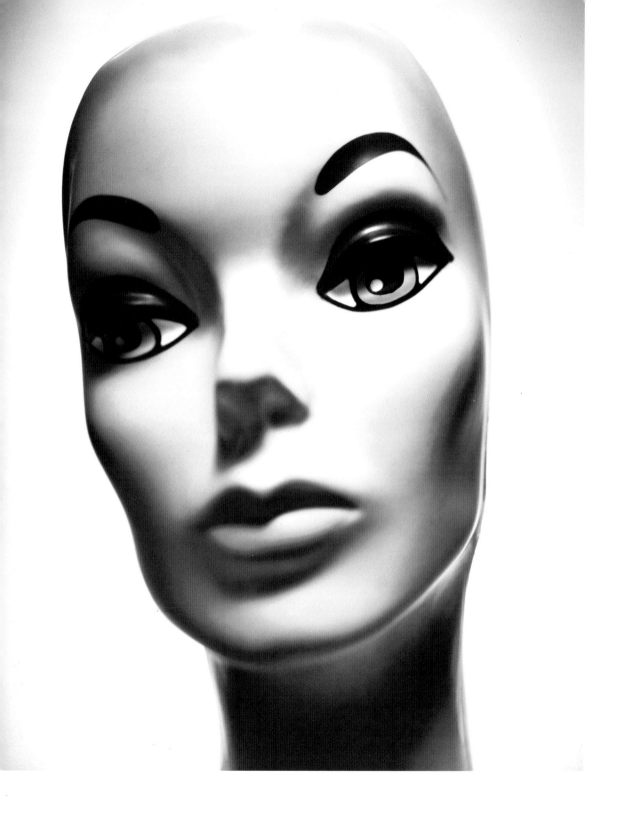

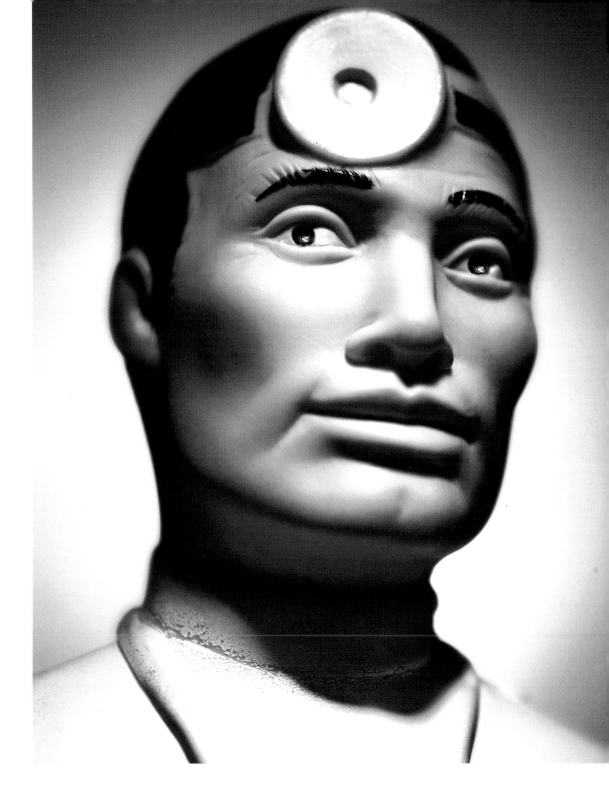

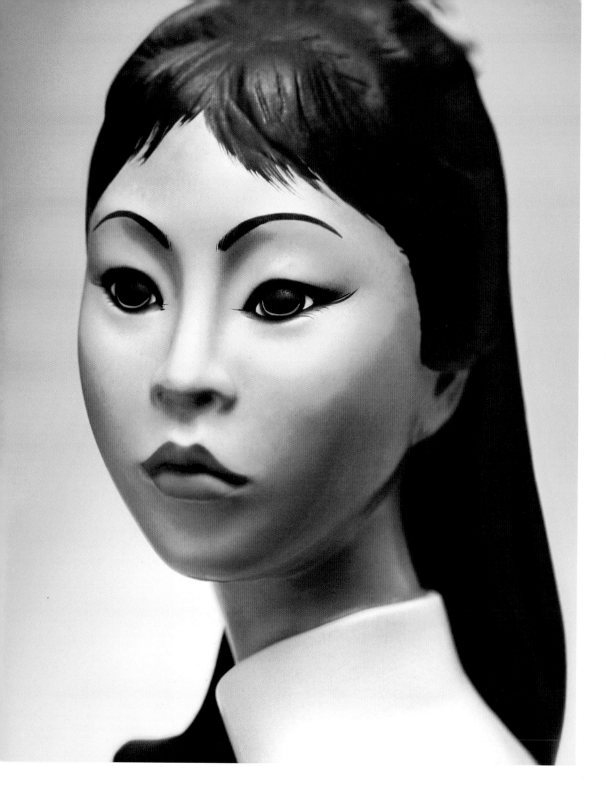

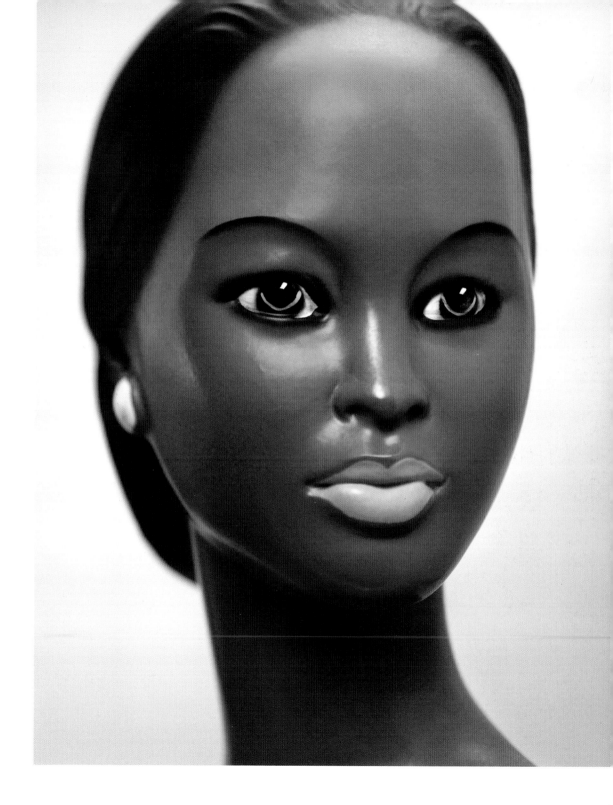

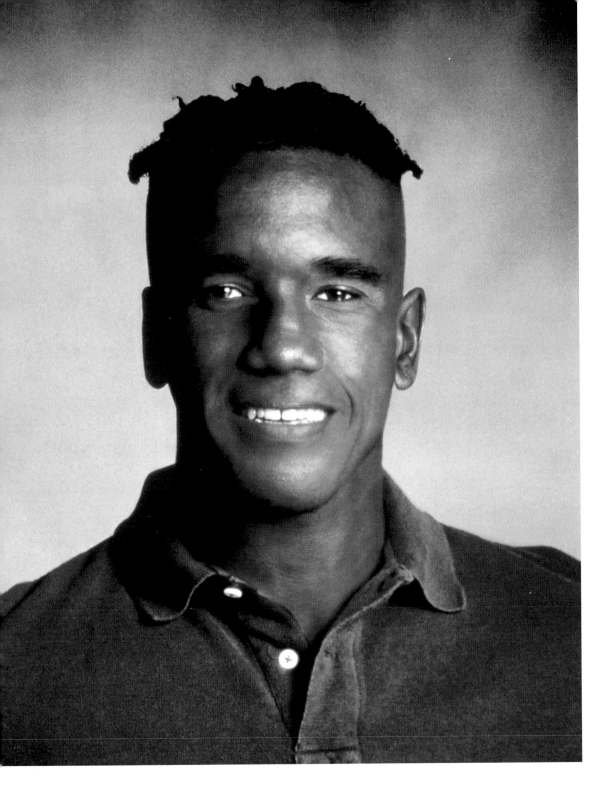

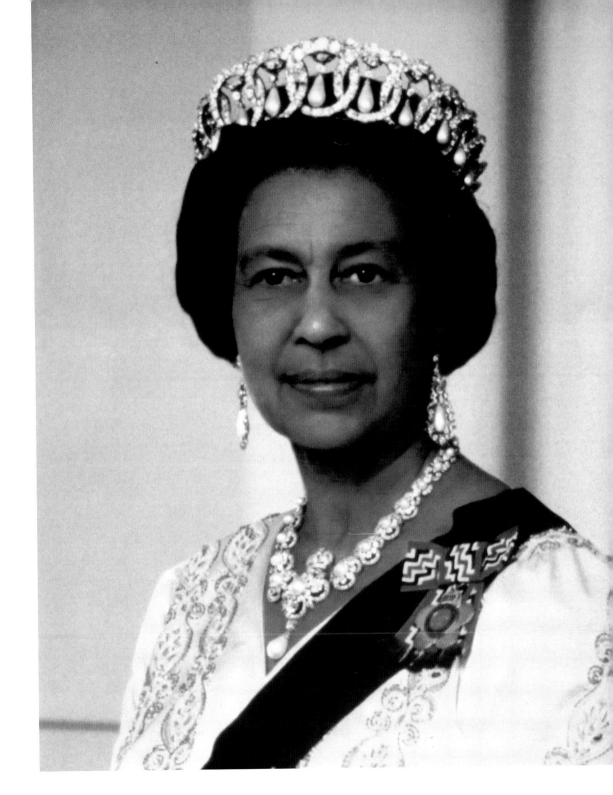

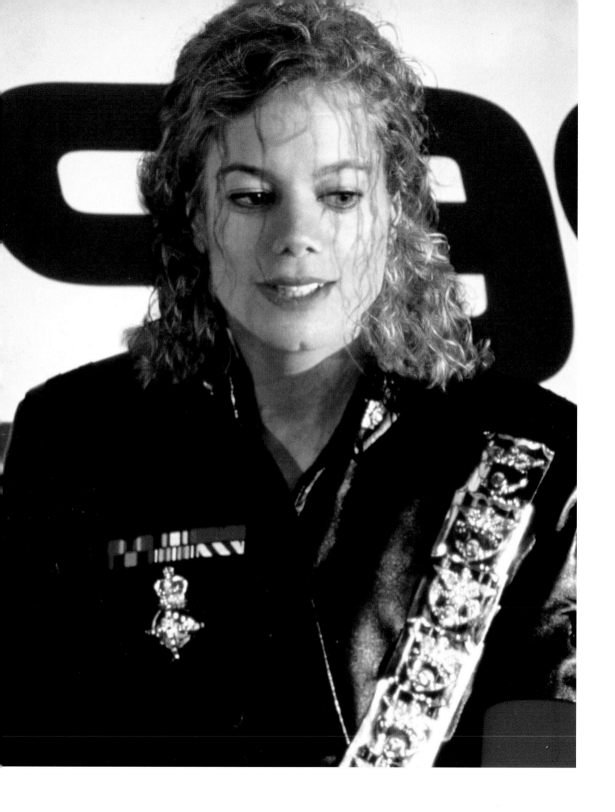

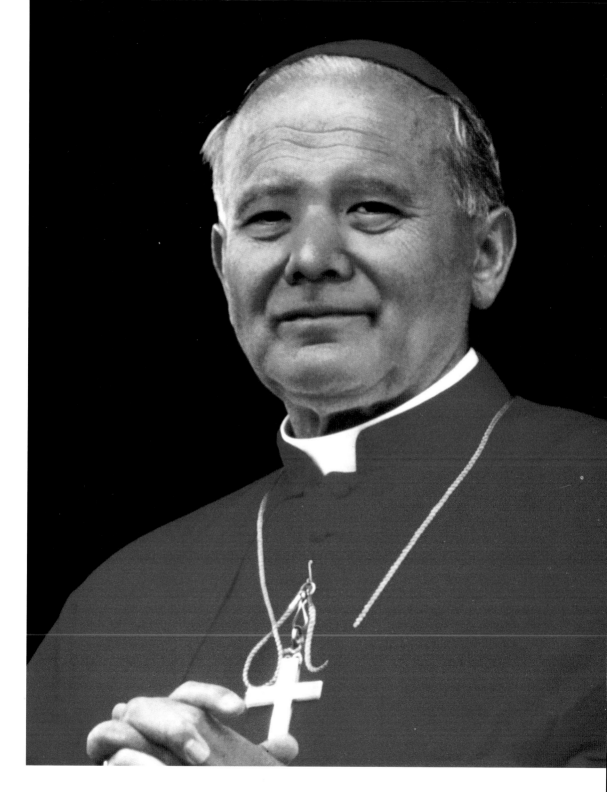

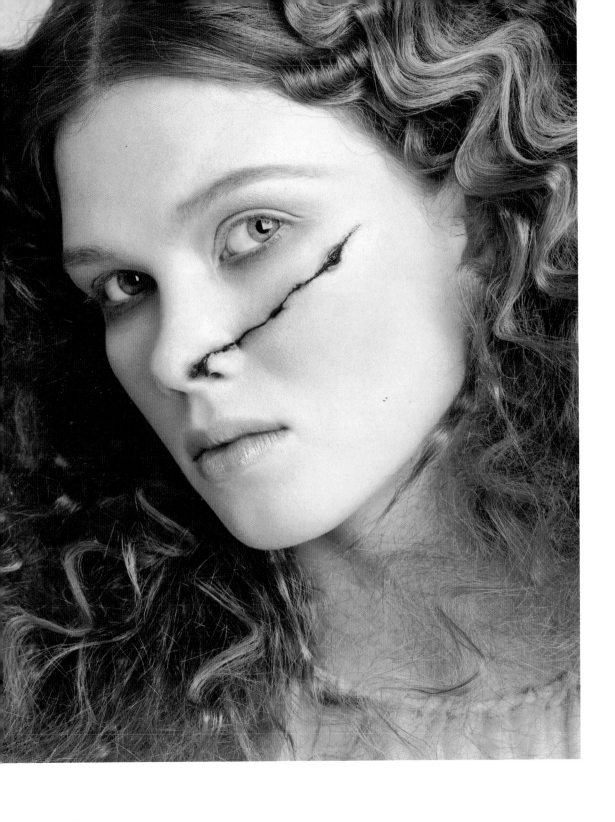

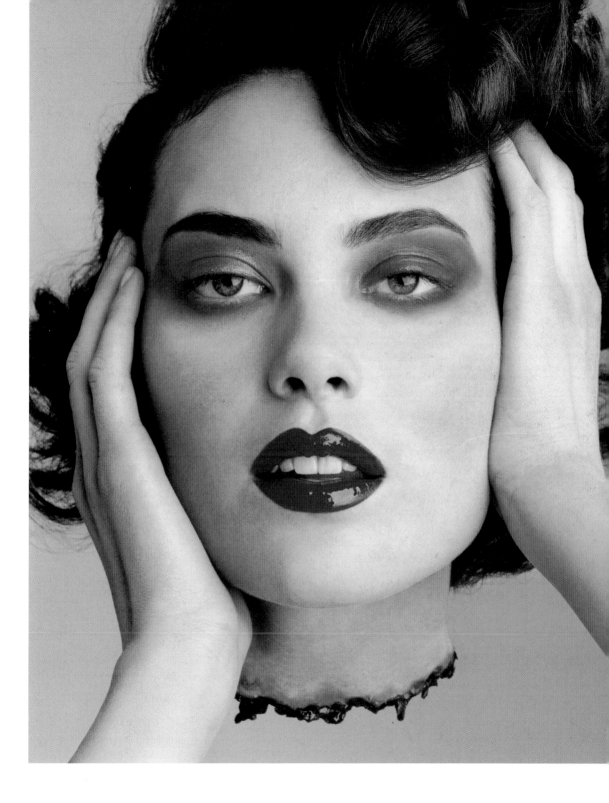

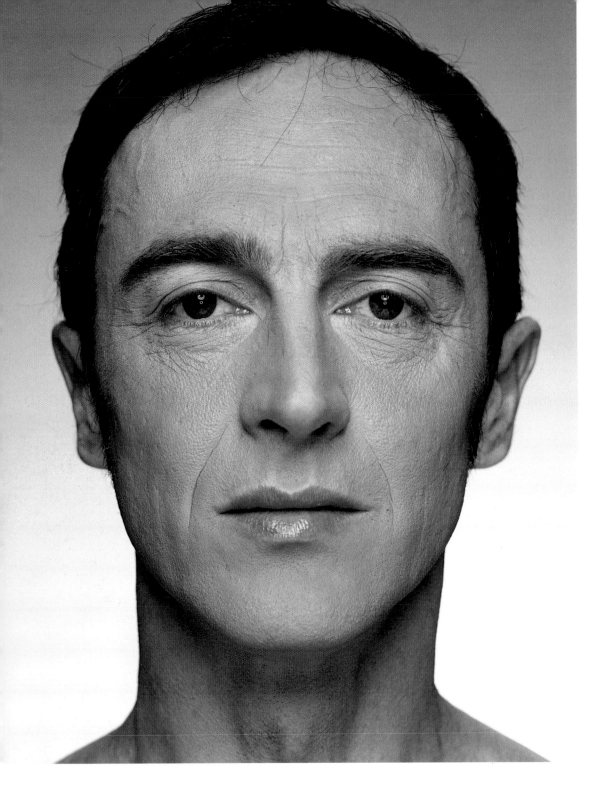

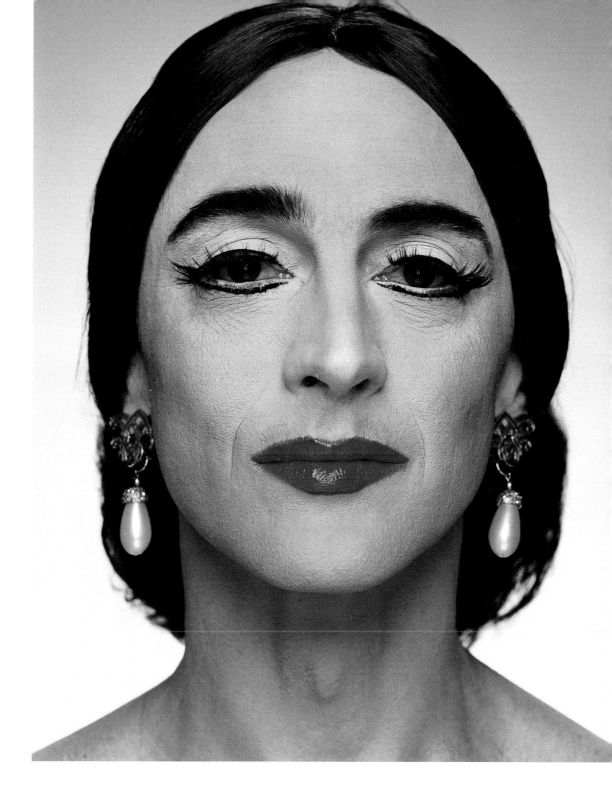

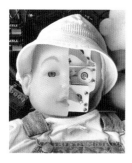

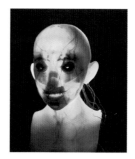

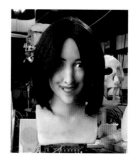

BIT (BABY IT), 2000

Photograph

DESIGNER Chi Won

MANUFACTURER iRobot, Somerville, Massachusetts

PHOTOGRAPHY Peter Menzel

© 2000 Peter Menzel/Robo Sapiens

Photographer Peter Menzel documented robot designs from around the world in his book, *Robo Sapiens: Evolution of a New Species*. Shown here is a dissected prototype for what later became My Real Baby, a Hasbro toy put to market in 2000. Lifelike skin is layered over a mechanical interior.

SECOND- AND THIRD-GENERATION FACE ROBOTS

Photographs, 2000

DESIGNERS Professors and student researchers of the Hara Kobayashi Laboratory, Science University of Tokyo

PROGRAM LEADERS Fumio Hara and Hiroshi Kobayashi

PHOTOGRAPHY © 2000 Peter Menzel/Robo Sapiens

The "face robot" is a research robot that may someday act as an interface between people and machines (such as a bank ATM) or as a companion for children or the elderly.

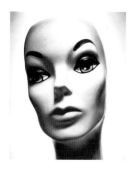

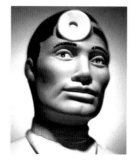

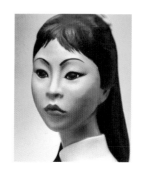

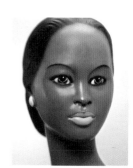

THE PORTRAIT SERIES, 2000

Photographs

ART DIRECTOR Charles S. Anderson, b. 1958

PHOTOGRAPHY Aaron Dimmel, b. 1974

Charles S. Anderson Design Co./CSA Images, Minneapolis

Designer and art director Charles Anderson has constructed an enormous stock of original photographs of plastic objects, including hundreds of portraits of figurines. The photographer, Aaron Dimmel, brings the camera in close to give these small objects a human scale and psychological presence, effects that conflict with their obvious artificiality.

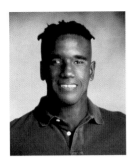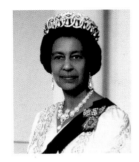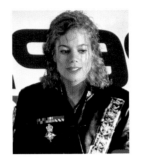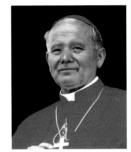

BLACK ARNOLD, BLACK QUEEN,
WHITE MICHAEL, ASIAN POPE, 1993
Photographs
DESIGN *Colors* magazine

Colors magazine published these digitally altered photographs
of international celebrities in its 1993 issue on race. The black
queen was especially controversial. Software programs such as
PhotoShop enable designers to manipulate our understanding of
photographic realities and falsehoods.

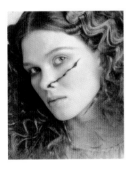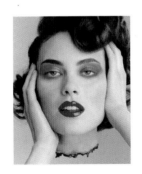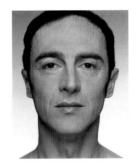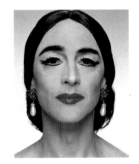

SCAR, HEADLESS, 2000
Photographs
PHOTOGRAPHY Phil Poynter, b. 1973
MAKEUP AND SPECIAL EFFECTS
Eileen Kastner-Delago, McKinny Macartney
RETOUCHING Colin Hume, The Shoemakers

JOHN KELLY, 2001
Photographs
PHOTOGRAPHY Martin Schoeller
ARTIST John Kelly
HAIR AND MAKEUP Bobby Miller

Performance artist John Kelly transforms himself into various
personalities, using sound, movement, music, and miming as well
as costumes and makeup to project such identities as the diva,
the artist, the pop star, and the gay man.

COOPER-HEWITT
NATIONAL DESIGN MUSEUM
SMITHSONIAN INSTITUTION

LAURENCE KING PUBLISHING

sk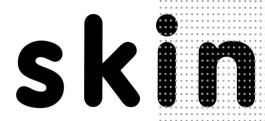in

SURFACE

SUBSTANCE

+

DESIGN

ELLEN LUPTON

With essays by
JENNIFER TOBIAS
ALICIA IMPERIALE
GRACE JEFFERS
RANDI MATES

Published in 2002 by Laurence King Publishing Ltd
71 Great Russell Street
London WC1B 3BP
Tel: +44 20 7430 8850
Fax: +44 20 7430 8880
e-mail: enquiries@laurenceking.co.uk
www.laurenceking.co.uk

A catalogue record for this book is available
from the British Library.

ISBN 1-85669-306-6

Printed and bound in China

contents

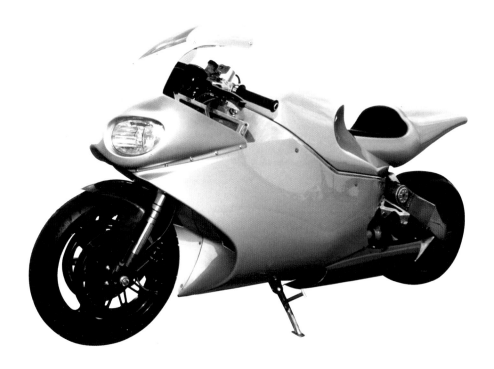

Y2K MOTORCYCLE, 2000

Carbon fiber, aluminum

DESIGNER Ted McIntyre, II, b. 1955

MANUFACTURER Marine Turbine Technologies, Louisiana

This hand-fabricated, limited-production motorcycle is the world's first turbine bike. Inventor/designer Ted McIntyre wanted to build a bike incorporating the same super-powerful engine used in helicopters. Rather than adapt existing body elements to the turbine, McIntyre designed and built the bike around the engine, creating a protective exoskeleton whose contours reflect the massive machinery inside. It is the world's fastest production motorcycle; it can reach speeds exceeding 250 mph and accelerates from 0–227 mph in less than fifteen seconds.

Skin, the complex membrane that holds the body together, also embraces the full spectrum of design today—from product to architecture, fashion, and media. Petra Blaisse, Nicholas Grimshaw, Hella Jongerius, Greg Lynn, and many other designers and architects are exploring new technologies, materials, and the exoskeletal qualities of the object. Cooper-Hewitt, National Design Museum curator Ellen Lupton, as ever, has her finger on the pulse of contemporary design, and I thank her for conceiving and designing this fascinating anthology of essays, images, and metaphors. My thanks, too, to everyone at Cooper-Hewitt and beyond who have made Skin possible.

PAUL WARWICK THOMPSON
Director
COOPER-HEWITT
NATIONAL DESIGN MUSEUM
SMITHSONIAN INSTITUTION

ACKNOWLEDGMENTS

ELLEN LUPTON
Curator of Contemporary Design
COOPER-HEWITT
NATIONAL DESIGN MUSEUM
SMITHSONIAN INSTITUTION

Many people and institutions helped create this book and the exhibition it accompanies. Numerous designers, photographers, firms, and manufacturers participated in the project, sharing their work and ideas. Their talents and resources made this project possible.

The National Design Museum's Board of Trustees generously supported the Skin project through the August Heckscher Exhibition Fund. Our gratitude goes to Kathleen B. Allaire (Chair), Arthur Ross (Vice Chair), Jorge L. Batista, Agnes Bourne, William Drenttel, Anne B. Ehrenkranz, Alice Gottesman, Paul K. Herzan, Harvey M. Krueger, Elaine La Roche, Jeffrey T. Leeds, Barbara A. Mandel, Nancy Marks, Richard Meier, Kenneth B. Miller, Maureen Miskovic, Enid W. Morse, Jon W. Rotenstreich, Donald H. Siskind, Richard M. Smith, Joan K. Davidson (honorary), Paul Warwick Thompson, *ex officio*, Sheila P. Burke, *ex officio*, and Lawrence M. Small, *ex officio*.

The exhibition received in-kind donations and crucial installation expertise from Pucci International, Wilsonart International, Lonseal, and Dynamic Systems; Cooper-Hewitt, National Design Museum thanks these corporations for their invaluable support.

The book was underwritten by the Andrew W. Mellon Foundation.

The exhibition was designed by Architecture Research Office (ARO), who embraced the challenge of displaying contemporary design in the historic Andrew Carnegie Mansion. It has been a pleasure to work with partners Adam Yarinsky and Stephen Cassell and their magnificent staff, especially Elizabeth Huck and Rosalyne Shieh.

The entire staff of Cooper-Hewitt, National Design Museum helped create Skin. Appreciation goes to everyone who contributed to the project's content, design, production, administration, development, marketing, maintenance, security, and educational programming. Above all, I am grateful to Paul Warwick Thompson, who enthusiastically supported the project when he joined the museum as director in early 2001, and to Susan Yelavich, Assistant Director of Public Programs, who helped shape the project from its inception. The leadership of these individuals has been indispensable.

Special thanks is directed to several key people at the museum: Elizabeth Johnson, editor, for refining the content of this book; Caroline Baumann, Development Director, and Jeffrey McCartney, Contracting Officer, for their unflagging efforts with exhibition and product development; Steven Langehough, Associate Registrar, for organizing the shipping of objects; Kristin Carvell and Jennifer Northrop in the Communications Department, for their insightful work in promoting the exhibition to the press and public; Dorothy Dunn, Head of Education, for her oversight of the project's relationship to all the museum's audiences; and Jennifer Brundage, Monica Hampton, and Mei Mah, for conceiving and implementing an exciting array of educational programs. Finally, extreme gratitude is owed to Lindsay Stamm Shapiro, Head of Exhibitions; Jen Roos and Alicia Cheng, Co-Directors of Design; and Jocelyn Groom, Scott Wilhelme, Linda Branning Doherty, Yve Ludwig, and the museum's full design and exhibitions staff, whose skills and talents helped create a safe, beautiful, and functional environment for Skin.

This publication reflects the museum's ongoing collaboration with Princeton Architectural Press. Special thanks goes to my editor, Mark Lamster, whose sense of language is both disciplined and generous, and to Kevin Lippert, publisher, who has been issuing important books on architecture and design for twenty years.

A wonderful team of writers provided essays for the book, including Alicia Imperiale, Grace Jeffers, Jennifer Tobias, and Randi Mates. In addition, they each helped shape the content of the exhibition in key ways. I am proud to count these women among my friends and collaborators.

My curatorial assistant, Kristina Kaufman, provided research for the book and exhibition and maintained endless contact with designers around the world while always coming up with exciting new objects and designers for consideration; I would never have survived the project without her.

Elke Gasselseder contributed her visual talent and technical expertise to the production of this book as well as to the research, editing, and design of video presentations for the exhibition. Kenneth Reinhard composed original music for the exhibition's multimedia components, providing an ideal aural counterpart to the project's visual themes.

My intern Kory Rogers, a student in Cooper-Hewitt's graduate program in the history of design and the decorative arts in Washington, D.C., covered key territory in my research on skin. Meagan Searing, a student in the same graduate program, helped inspire the idea for Skin with her own research on the design of cosmetics. I also thank my students and colleagues at Maryland Institute, College of Art, for their ideas and support; special thanks goes to Claudia Matzko and Jenna Zilincar.

Lucy Fellowes has been my trusted friend and colleague for nearly a decade at the museum; I will continue to seek her guidance as she embarks on new adventures.

My family is a constant source of pleasure and inspiration. My love goes out to Jay, Ruby, and Abbott; to Mary Jane and Ken; to Bill and Shirley; to Michelle, Anwar, and Layla; and to Julia, Ken, and all their children.

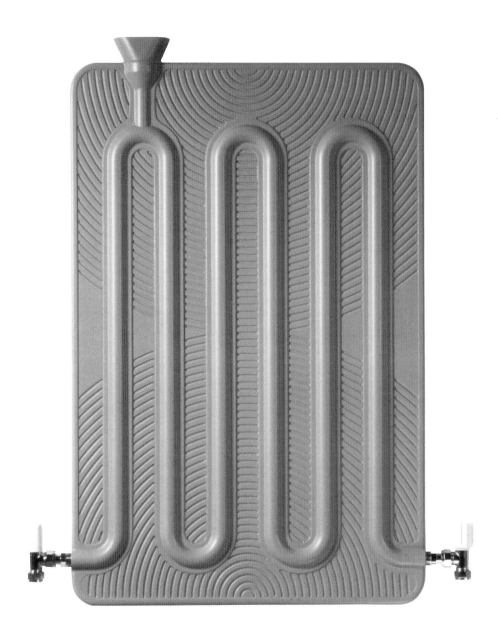

HOT-WATER BOTTLE, 1999
Prototype for radiator, painted wood
DESIGNER Emma Quickenden, b. 1976
Kingston University, United Kingdom
PHOTOGRAPHY Malcolm Kennard

This prototype is for a rubber radiator that would encase
metal plumbing pipes inside a resilient skin, exchanging
a harsh industrial vernacular for softer forms. The circular
grooves in the surface resemble stylized, standardized
fingerprints. The object—modeled after a hot-water bottle—
evokes the antiseptic comforts of nursing care as well as
tactility and warmth, reflecting the overtly technological,
clinically erotic attitude of the new design organics.

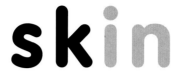

sk in

NEW DESIGN ORGANICS

ELLEN LUPTON

SKIN is a multilayered, multipurpose organ that shifts from thick to thin, tight to loose, lubricated to dry, across the landscape of the body. Skin, a knowledge-gathering device, responds to heat and cold, pleasure and pain. It lacks definitive boundaries, flowing continuously from the exposed surfaces of the body to its internal cavities. It is both living and dead, a self-repairing, self-replacing material whose exterior is senseless and inert while its inner layers are flush with nerves, glands, and capillaries. Contemporary designers approach the surfaces of products and buildings as similarly complex, ambiguous forms. Manufactured skins are richly responsive substances that modulate the meaning, function, and dimension of things.

In the 1940s and 1950s, organic forms and materials provided designers with a humanist vocabulary that affirmed society's place within the natural world. By the end of the century, a new organicism had emerged, as nature itself was transformed by a host of technologies. In the 1990s, plants and animals with altered DNA were dispersed through the global food market. The successful cloning of a sheep in Scotland in 1997 plunged a science-fiction fantasy into practice. In the summer of 2000, the human genome was mapped—a competitive venture between government and private enterprise—laying bare new terrains for medical science and economic conquest. In the mid-1990s, the new field of tissue engineering emerged, charged with the manufacture of human organs. While complete hearts, lungs, and kidneys cannot yet be generated from living cells, skin is already a viable medical product, grown in laboratories.

During the 1990s, cosmetic surgeries and products were marketed to an expanding and unembarrassed public, as many people came to see surgical alteration as no more objectionable than diet and exercise.[1] Consumption of breast implants and liposuction doubled between 1997 and 2000. The demand for nonsurgical dermatological procedures soared during the late 1990s as well. Injections of fat or collagen are used to temporarily fill shallow lines and acne scars. Chemical peels remove the outermost layer of the epidermis, erasing sun damage and other blemishes by exposing a fresh layer of cells. Cosmeceuticals, a rapidly growing over-the-counter product category, deliver low concentrations of acids and other chemicals, and claim to repair skin at the biological level.[2] Botox injections allow a small dose of the toxin that causes botulism to paralyze selected facial muscles, easing wrinkles caused by habitual frowning and eyebrow-raising—the number of Botox procedures performed in the United States doubled between 1999 and 2000, having risen sixteenfold since 1997.[3]

A sense of horror as well as enthusiasm accompanies these developments. Environmentalists warn against an ecosystem unhinged by genetically altered species, while bioethicists condemn human cloning and envision a society dominated by a self-replicating elite.[4] At the same time that humanity risks reduction to a genetic code, concerns are arising about the potential humanity of machines, as seen in films such as Steven Spielberg's A.I. (2001). Scientific research is increasingly motivated by profit and loss—life-saving drugs and newly identified DNA sequences are patented and sold for financial gain, while unchecked diseases devastate local and international economies. Cosmetic surgeries are consumed by the privileged few—anxious to prolong the attributes of youth into lives ever-lengthened by medical services—even as the lack of basic health care and sanitation shortens the life spans of millions around the world.

Designed objects and spaces inhabit this rapidly transforming arena, where surging fears and ambitions fuel scientific discovery and stimulate the creation and consumption of new technologies. Design reflects and shapes our understanding of the world; it is both symptom and cure. As a practice embedded in the fabric of technology and commerce, design responds critically to the very culture it serves to replicate and extend.

1 Gina Bellafante, "In This Bare-It-All Age, Bikinis are Back," New York Times, 5 June 2001.
2 Statistics reported by the American Society for Aesthetic Plastic Surgery, 2001.
3 For a description of cosmeceuticals, see Nicholas Perricone, The Wrinkle Cure (Emmaus, PA: Rodale, 2000).
4 On the commercial development of the human genome, see Wil S. Hylton, "Who Owns this Body?" Esquire, June 2001, 103–11. On the ethics of cloning, see Dr. Ian Wilmut, "The Rights and Wrongs of Cloning Humans," Twice 2:1 (1998): 3–15.

The rise of digital media over the past decade has changed the practice of design, providing tools for making objects and buildings that resemble living creatures—modeled with complex curves and forms—while remaining distinctly artificial. This new organicism has taken shape most aggressively across the surface of things. The primacy of the skeleton has given way to the primacy of skin. Surfaces have acquired depth, becoming dense, complex substances equipped with their own identities and behaviors. New materials react to light, heat, touch, and mechanical stress. Translucency and mutability have replaced transparency and permanence. The outer envelope has detached from the interior volume. Flexible membranes are embedded with digital and mechanical networks. Thin planes of material are folded, warped, or pumped with air to become load-bearing structures. Industrial skins have assumed a life of their own. It is a life whose pedigree, however, is more alien than human.

SKIN IS BOTH DEAD AND ALIVE. The thin outer layer, the epidermis, consists of strata of cells that migrate toward the surface, where they compact into a layer of dead material. Skin's protective function relies on the inertness of this outer surface. Mark C. Taylor, whose 1997 book *Hiding* is a commentary on the culture of skin, writes, "Death, like life, is not a momentary event but is an ongoing process whose traces line the body. At the point where I make contact with the world, I am always already dead."[5]

This convergence of life and death also structures our relationship to the object world. Skin, hair, and nails are products of the body, continuously sloughed off and renewed. Hair is part of the skin, its cells generated deep within the living dermis and pushed upward into shafts of protein, emerging across the body's landscape as a thicket of dead blades. Skin is connected to our bodies yet also alien, marking the exterior, the end of our selves. It is a screen on which we can watch the body's amazing ability to heal itself while also witnessing its inevitable collapse.

Many of the earliest technologies were created to supplement the inadequacies of this natural envelope. The first shelters and the first garments, made from animal skins, protected humans against hostile climates. Today, military and aerospace technologies are being used to extend the

5. Mark C. Taylor, Hiding (Chicago: University of Chicago Press, 1997), 13.

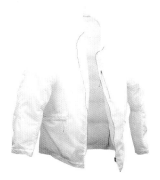

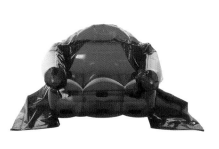

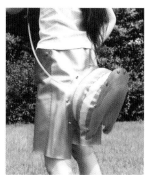

body's tolerance of extreme temperatures. In Italy, Corpo Nove has created the hyperinsulated Absolute Zero jacket, lined with the cloudlike substance Aerogel, one of the lightest materials on Earth. The Cooling System jacket, also by Corpo Nove, is plumbed with plastic tubes that carry water across the body, as used in space suits. CP Company has produced a series of raincoats that inflate to become chairs, tents, or mattresses, while the Tokyo partnership ixilab has created prototypes for garments that are also stools, floor mats, or storage units. By providing survival gear for the urban nomad or the eco-tourist, these products suggest a culture where danger and disaster coexist with leisure and entertainment, animating the surface of experience.

Such projects recall the Pop movement of the 1960s, with its embrace of portable structures and synthetic materials. Pierre Cardin introduced his vinyl minidress in 1968, using a sculptural, preformed fabric made by American Cyanamid—an artificial skin with its own dimensional markings. In contrast with the implied optimism of Cardin's Pop couture, the vinyl and PVC fashions of Walter van Beirendonck are apocalyptic party clothes. The shiny surface of a 1998 red synthetic suit bubbles with protrusions, like scales on a futuristic dragon. On the runway, models danced in gas masks, implying the presence of a toxic process.

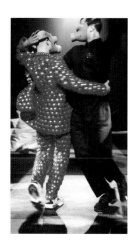

NYLON MINIDRESSES, 1968
DESIGNER Pierre Cardin, b. 1922
PHOTOGRAPHY Yoshi Takata

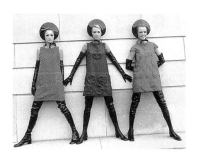

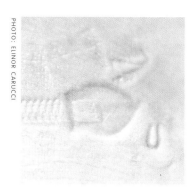

PHOTO: ELINOR CARUCCI

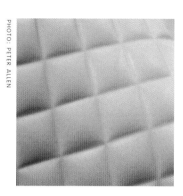

PHOTO: PETER ALLEN

6 Chris Hables Gray, ed., *The Cyborg Handbook* (New York: Routledge, 1995).

Like skin, design performs at the intersection of life and death, body and product. Human beings, using objects to survive and conquer, rely on the world of things, merging their own identities with the objects they use. Photographer Elinor Carucci, whose pictures appear throughout this book, has used her camera to reveal intimate relations between skin and everyday industrial products, from lipstick and pantyhose to zippers, bras, and buttons. Industrial designers Carla Murray and Peter Allen propose more grotesque conjoinings of bodies and consumer goods in their project Skinthetic (2001), which predicts the grafting of brand identities into living tissue. Skin is the surface where bodies and products merge.

In modern civilization, dependence on technologies has become absolute. From birth, the human organism is enmeshed in an infrastructure that controls and delivers food, water, light, climate, health care, and entertainment. This modern creature of comfort has become a cyborg, a living thing whose functions are enhanced by technology.[6] Monstrous beings come to mind, along with everyday pacemakers, hearing aids, prosthetic limbs, and even pagers, cell phones, and wristwatches.

Our increasing dependence on the artificial is not without anxiety, a phenomenon most vividly expressed in science fiction. In *Star Trek: First Encounter* (1996), the leader of the villainous army of Borg consists of a dis-embodied mechanical nervous system covered with glossy, translucent skin—she is a head and shoulders with no body. She descends into a metal gown whose connective fasteners bite down into her soft, lubricated flesh. The hero of the same film has a nightmare recalling his seduction by the Borg; in his dream, a spiderlike mechanical probe pushes out through the

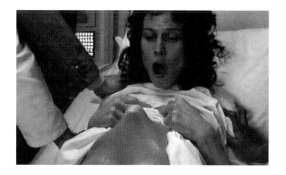

ALIENS, 1986
DIRECTOR
James Cameron
WRITERS
James Cameron, David Giler,
Walter Hill
COURTESY OF
20th Century Fox

elastic skin of his cheek, searching bluntly from behind the soft layers before cutting through with its sharp prongs.

The fear of invasion from within the body drives many depictions of beings from outer space. In the *Alien* films, the enemy is most frightening when it occupies a human host, incubating inside the body before erupting through the abdomen or chest. A dream sequence in *Aliens* (1986) shows Sigourney Weaver—prone on a hospital bed—watching with horror as a mechanical-looking object probes upward through her belly, threatening a hideous birth. The clinical setting heightens the shock of the scene, with its threat of physical helplessness and humiliation.

David Cronenberg's *Videodrome* (1983) conjoins the body and machinery in reverse: here, inanimate objects pulse with life. First a video-cassette, then a television and VCR, swell, buckle, and moan, their plastic surfaces heaving with morbid sexuality. The screen of the TV bulges out-ward, filled with a video image of Deborah Harry's half-open, lipsticked mouth, which threatens to engulf the shocked but willing hero, played by James Woods. Later, a hand and gun press through the elastic surface of the screen, turning into a slippery, engorged hybrid of flesh and machine.

Like cinema, design offers imaginative responses to the conver-gence of life and technology, sometimes celebrating the relationship and other times recoiling from it. Contemporary objects and spaces are cloaked in surfaces that have been enhanced, simulated, or engineered, surfaces that masquerade as other materials, surfaces where the physical and the virtual, the real and the imagined, collide. Hard surfaces look soft, and soft surfaces

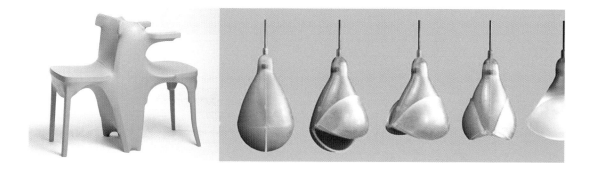

look hard. Wood is sealed inside of resin; smooth planes are rippled, bubbled, or scarred with digital imagery; luminescent fabrics, gels, and plywoods glow with preternatural life.

Jurgen Bey's Kokon series, initiated in 1997, encloses traditional wooden furnishings inside a tight wrapping of PVC. The familiar, humanly scaled limbs of the found objects press through a grossly artificial skin. In Kokon Double Chair, two chairs are bound, back to back, like lovers held hostage in a dysfuntional embrace. Moorhead & Moorhead's Rubber Lamp No. 5 has a flexible shade of translucent rubber that peels open to direct the flow of light, evoking the alien pods from the films *Invasion of the Body Snatchers* (1956, 1978).

Organic design vocabularies—from the ecstasies of baroque ornament to mid-twentieth-century biomorphism—have always gestured toward the erotic, suggesting the curves and movements of the human body. In contemporary design, eroticism is present yet kept at a distance, handled with rubber gloves. The fulfillment of desire and the satisfaction of touch are blunted by protective layers of material. Clothed in latex, vinyl, rubber, or resin, sensual forms are rendered clinical. When love and fear are necessary bedfellows, the plush, dimly lit boudoir gives way to the bright, wipeable surfaces of the laboratory and lavatory.

EVA CHAIR, 2000
Beech plywood, lacquer, steel, polyurethane foam, plastic
DESIGNERS
Simo Heikkilä, b. 1946
Yrjö Wiherheimo, b. 1941
MANUFACTURER
Klaessons, Sweden

The Eva chair is a plane of curved plywood hovering within a steel frame. The arms and legs supporting Eva's mysterious body, however, are detailed in a vocabulary that is more therapeutic than erotic. The armrests resemble handles on medical equipment or sports gear, while the chair legs are tipped with elongated sheaths of protective plastic.

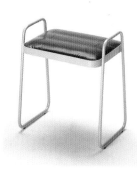
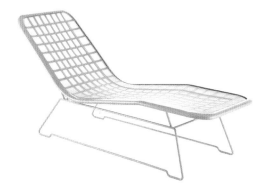

TechnoGel, developed for the health-care industry in the 1970s, typically is used in wheelchairs or hospital beds, supporting the body with minimal friction. Designers have adopted this soft polyurethane material for its cool yet fleshy texture—it is said to have the consistency of human fat.[7] The Tino stool (1999), designed by Alessandro Scarpellini Piva, is padded with TechnoGel; the armrests rise up like bathroom grips or the side rails of a walker. Werner Aisslinger's Soft chaise is an indoor/outdoor lounge chair. A web of nylon straps is padded with a seamless slab of TechnoGel, protecting its user's skin from unsightly impressions while providing an ideal resting place for invalids and sunbathers.

Latex is another material whose clinical functionality cloaks the eroticism of contemporary design. Matthieu Manche has created latex garments that propose links among multiple wearers and the proliferation of body parts. He uses the material of self-protection to suggest the merging and elaboration, rather than the separation and containment, of bodies. Tonita Abeyta's Sensate is a line of latex undergarments—some equipped with built-in male and female condoms—that aim to transform the tools of sexual hygiene into alluring fashion objects.

7 Chee Pearlman, "From Bike Seat to Chaise: Is Gel the New Black?" *New York Times*, 12 April 2001.

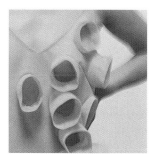

P73

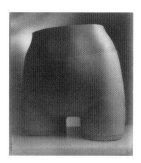

P74

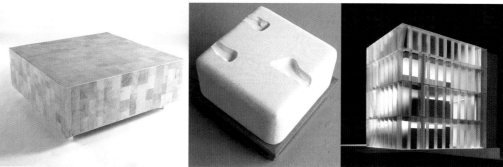

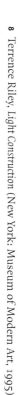

8 Terrence Riley, Light Construction (New York: Museum of Modern Art, 1995).

In furniture designed by Elizabeth Paige Smith, the outer layer becomes a viscous medium. Her Cube table (1998) is a built-up block of balsa wood interred in a deep coat of resin. While conventional finishes heighten the visual texture of wood, Smith's milky skin provides a palpable layer of protection. Timothy McLoughlin's 2001 *Ottoman (Customized for K. Fischer)* is a pristine white volume that has been physically violated. Upholstered in fragile white fabric, the surface of the stool appears gouged with a path of footprints. McLoughlin has inserted rubber castings of footprints into the stool's foam padding, suturing them into place with the care of a surgeon and covering the scars with flocking. McLoughlin's *Ottoman* uses modernism's white cube—archetype of the silent, static object—as the stage for a temporal narrative.

Smith's thick coat of resin brings an element of time to her Cube table as well, slowing down our view of the natural surface. Terrence Riley describes how materials serve to delay and materialize the passage of light in his 1995 book *Light Construction*. Contemporary architects have exchanged the transparent skins of early modernism for physically present, semi-opaque surfaces. Buildings are clothed in multiple skins that trap and reflect light, from translucent marble to double layers of glass.[8]

Temporal change animates the skin of Gluckman Mayner's Helmut Lang Tokyo showroom (2001), which pulses with shifting light effects. Composed of translucent glass and LCD panels, the store's gridded facade is 60 centimeters deep, functioning as a vast showcase and a field of dynamic light patterns, transforming from opaque to transparent to translucent over

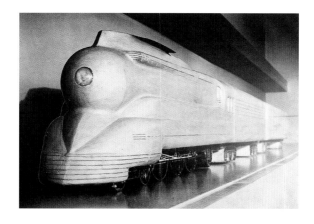

S-1 LOCOMOTIVE, 1936
Photograph, clay scale model
DESIGNER
Raymond Loewy, 1893–1986
COLLECTION OF Cooper-Hewitt,
National Design Museum,
Smithsonian Institution,
1937-58-6
Raymond Loewy's streamlined
locomotives were icons of aero-
dynamic styling.

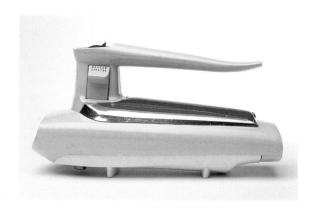

PORTABLE HAND MIXER
c. 1955
Plastic, metal
MANUFACTURER
General Electric, U.S.A.
COLLECTION OF Cooper-Hewitt,
National Design Museum,
Smithsonian Institution
In the 1950s, everything from a
kitchen implement to a Cadillac
was enclosed in a hard,
horizontally elongated skin.

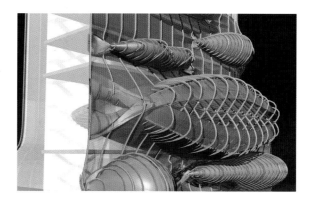

EYEBEAM COMPETITION:
DETAIL OF BUILDING
SKIN
Digital rendering, 2001
DESIGNER Greg Lynn, b. 1964
Greg Lynn FORM, Santa Monica
Architect Greg Lynn uses 3d-
modeling software to create
forms shaped by dynamic
forces.

the course of a day. The glass facade can either reveal or conceal the contents of the building; it functions like a multilayered, three-dimensional cinema screen, whose narrative is populated by the merchandise, the customer, the concrete shell within, or the skin of the glowing white box itself.

Greg Lynn confronts temporality by stretching the skin of architecture into the dimension of time. According to his concept "animate form," digital design tools plunge three-dimensional structures into a space that ripples with currents of force. Lynn writes that in place of a neutral abstract space, "the context of design becomes an active abstract space that directs form within a current of forces that can be stored as information in the shape of the form." The undulating skins of Lynn's "blobs" record the object's passage through fields of pressure.[9]

The idea that the shape of an object can refer to its own motion through a fluid medium is linked to the origins of the industrial design profession. In the 1920s and 1930s, Raymond Loewy, Norman Bel Geddes, and other pioneering industrial designers drew upon engineering principles that had been employed in naval and aeronautical design since the nineteenth century, when the curved shells of ships and zeppelins were designed to minimize drag as vessels push through air or water. In the 1930s designers employed aerodynamic forms to impress the image of speed and modernity on the bodies of cars, trains, and planes as well as on such stationary objects as toasters, staplers, and pencil sharpeners. The teardrop became an icon of 1930s modernism.[10]

The early industrial designers created skins for mechanical devices that enclosed their working innards inside smooth, streamlined shells. These gleaming surfaces became the interface between body and product, protecting the mechanisms from water, dirt, and interference from the user. Documenting his work in the manner of a cosmetic surgeon, Raymond Loewy promoted his achievement through Before and After photographs.[11]

While Loewy's skins aimed to conceal, product skins today are often transparent or translucent. The iMac (1997) revealed the electronic components of the computer through a candy-colored shell, providing visibility while maintaining the fundamental structure of the protective casing. Other industrial surfaces have become softer, more giving to the touch,

9 Greg Lynn, Animate Form (New York: Princeton Architectural Press, 1999) 11.
    See also Joseph Rosa, Folds, Blobs and Boxes: Architecture in the Digital Era (Pittsburgh: Heinz Architectural Center, Carnegie Museum of Art, 2001).
10 Donald J. Bush, The Streamlined Decade (New York: Braziller, 1975).
11 Raymond Loewy, Never Leave Well Enough Alone (New York: Simon and Schuster, 1951).

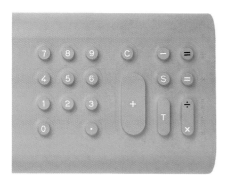

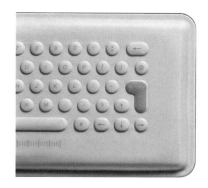

enhancing the object's creaturelike presence. Mario Bellini designed an adding machine for Olivetti in 1972, covering the keyboard in flesh-toned rubber. In 2001 the design firm IDEO published prototypes using ElekTex, a conductive fabric whose entire surface can sense the location and pressure of human touch: "It allows a product to have a skin that is flexible, that is itself a functioning, intelligent organ."[12]

Skins also mediate between users and products in the digital realm. The customized buttons and controls used in computer interfaces are known as skins. Thousands of skins can be downloaded from the Web, allowing users to create and exchange interfaces that are colored, coded, themed, and branded to suit individual whims. Avatars, the graphical personalities used to represent players in computer games, are also known as skins—they are the digital surfaces of invented personae. In 2001, the first feature film cast entirely with digital, photoreal human characters—Final Fantasy—was released. Such characters are created by imposing digital surfaces over wire-frame structures.

12 IDEO Europe, Fabrications (London: IDEO and ElectroTextiles, 2001), 67.

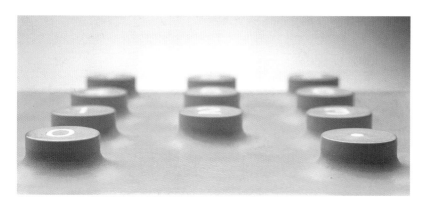

IN AN EDITORIAL in the *New York Times* (11 April 2001), Maureen Dowd commented on the use of bovine collagen as a "line filler" in dermatological procedures as well as an ingredient in numerous cosmetic potions and creams. As communicative diseases devastated livestock across Europe at the turn of the twenty-first century, cattle-based products could have fallen into disfavor. Yet the alien had already been invited in, and it is hard to banish such a charming guest. Dowd quotes dermatologist Patricia Wexler: "I've never had a patient ask about a kosher cow. I've never had a vegetarian model object to bovine collagen. I've never had an animal rights activist object to cows getting killed for collagen. When it comes to cosmetic matters, women have a 'Don't ask, don't tell me, please!' policy."

The substance of the body is under renovation. The arsenal of drugs, vaccines, and mechanical replacement parts developed during the twentieth century is now joined by the engineering of flesh itself. While living skin has become a commercially manufactured product, objects and buildings have come to resemble natural organisms. The barriers between body and product, self and other, nature and technology, are folding inward. The dense, luminous surfaces of contemporary objects—pulsing with hidden intelligence or taut with potential life—can be beautiful and disturbing, divine and grotestque. These industrial skins may be incubating something alien. They could be shielding us from invisible dangers or harboring the nascent growth of a predatory being. Everywhere, prophylactic skins slip into the space between people and things, forming seductive planes of contact as well as protective barriers, screens where image replaces tactility or where touch triggers a visual response—points of no entry or no return.

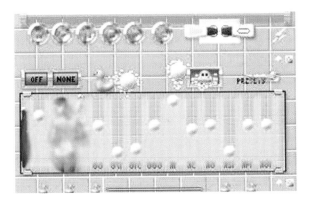

INTERFACE
SKIN, 2001

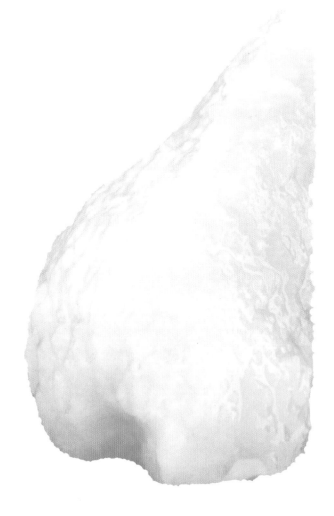

CARTILAGE NOSE, 1999

RESEARCHERS

Prasad V. Shastri and Ivan Martin

Massachusetts Institute of Technology

This nose was made by seeding a synthetic polymer scaffold with cartilage cells, which gradually replaced the polymer with engineered tissue, leaving behind a likeness of a human nose. The cells were obtained from the knee of a bovine calf. (Human cells may be easily obtained by nipping a microscopic sample of the cartilage in the ear and growing cells in a Petri dish.)

artificial
skin

JENNIFER TOBIAS

The 1973 sci-fi comedy *Sleeper* depicts a sleek, plastic-coated future that provides virtual sex, robotic dogs, and blobular vehicles. The film ends with an attempted cloning, in which doctors seek to reconstitute their dictator from only his nose. Fumbling over a body-shaped operating table, Woody Allen and Diane Keaton willfully botch the procedure and kidnap the nose, which is ultimately flattened by an oncoming steamroller, and reduced to an absurd silhouette.

Today, cloning is not a science-fiction fantasy but a technological fact. The laboratory production of skin grafts is an early triumph for the new fields of tissue engineering and regenerative medicine, which seek to manufacture living replacement parts for the human body. Working with tools ranging from polymer scaffolds and epidermal growth factors to cell "seeding," biotechnologists grow replacements for irretrievably damaged skin and are now making progress with tissues such as bone, valves, and cartilage. Skin is "cultured" in the lab, the mind, and the body.

Living skin consists of multiple layers, each in a constant state of synthesis and transformation. Skin appears early in the transformation from ovum to fetus. In the process of cellular differentiation that unfolds in the first phases of life, skin appears before the organs and structures it will contain. As cultural theorist Mark C. Taylor has pointed out, the complex systems of the body are generated from layers of skin. Cells form a hollow ball (blastomere) that subdivides into three dermal layers: the ectoderm, endoderm, and mesoderm. These layers generate the nerves, skin, internal organs, skeleton, connective tissue, muscles, and other systems. Taylor explains that "the body is, in effect, nothing but strata of skin in which interiority and exteriority are thoroughly convoluted."[1]

Skin, whether generated by the body or manufactured in a lab, is crucial as a barrier, container, and biochemical manufactory. Skin protects the body from infection and harmful radiation as well as mechanical and electrical forces. It is a heterogeneous, flexible container for our squirmy, curvy selves. Skin is also our largest organ: the dermis alone makes up 15 to 20 percent of body weight. Skin is necessary for maintaining body temperature and fluid balance. Some skin components synthesize growth factors and vitamins; others clean up cellular wastes.[2]

Natural skin also carries nerve endings, providing our sense of touch. Skin communicates emotional and physical states: it can blush and blanch,[3] get goose pimples and sweat, go blue with cold, red with anger, or metaphorically green with envy. Skin communicates in the form of pheromones, hormonal signals believed to be received by specialized cells in the nose. Emergency medics can quickly assess a person's physical state by squeezing a finger, noticing how quickly the skin "pinks up" after blood is momentarily withheld.[4]

Natural skin is composed of two layers. The skin we see and touch (the epidermis) is composed of cells called keratinocytes. The epidermis is generated by the dermis beneath. The bottom-most layer of epidermal cells migrate upward, die, compact, and slough off. These dead cells form the body's barrier to the outside world (the cells are glued together with lipids into a water-repellant layer). The epidermis also contains melanocytes

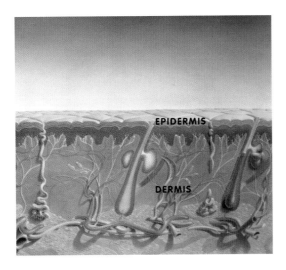

EPIDERMIS

DERMIS

(pigment cells bearing melanin), Langerhans cells (for immune response), macrophages (for cellular clean-up), and mast cells (for inflammatory response).

Skin differentiates across the body. The "thick-skinned" soles and palms lack sweat glands, and they build up layers of dead cells (calluses) in response to mechanical stress. Skin grows around our curves and cracks—in a lab, it will grow freely, even around itself, until it forms a ball or sac. Other areas are highly elastic, such as the skin over the elbow. Still others are packed with nerve cells and engorgeable capillaries.

Skin represents a transition between our outsides and insides. Where does the lip end and the mouth begin? Is a navel an "outie" or an "innie"? The ambiguous transition between inside and out is as plain as the nose on your face: skin is continuous over and into the nose, differentiating into nose-specific cells at some dark inner point (a transition almost more anatomical than biological).[5] Cartilage, the tissue giving shape to the nose and ears, is structurally similar to the surrounding skin. Both have a small variety of cell types and relatively low blood-vessel requirements, making them initial targets for tissue engineering.[6] The inside of the nose has hair, and the nose responds to temperature much like other hirsute areas, shivering to fluff the hairs and conserve heat. A passionate flaring of the nostrils is possible because of the flexible interaction of skin, cartilage, and muscle. This flexibility and the ability to partially regenerate also make the nose resilient after trauma.

The inner dermis is generally thicker than the epidermis. Its components—nerve cells, lymph and sweat glands, hair follicles, fibroblasts (which produce collagen), and blood vessels bearing oxygen (which keeps it all alive)—are suspended in a thicket of collagen cells (strandlike proteins with a mesh or scaffoldlike structure). Below the dermis lie fat, veins, arteries, and muscle. The dermis has two layers: hair follicles, glands, nerves, and vessels are distributed in an upper layer of thin collagen and elastic fibers, and the lower layer is made of thick collagen and elastic fibers. The elastic fibers allow skin to rebound when pressed. A vertebrate animal can have at least ten different kinds of collagen, each specialized for a particular tissue such as skin, tendon, ligament, blood vessels, or bone.[7]

If dermis is damaged, its original form cannot be regenerated by the body. Instead, scar collagen forms. Surviving epidermal cells migrate

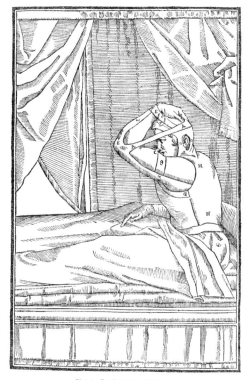

Fig. 63. *De Curtorum Chirurgia.*
Plate IX

from the edges of a wound to help heal it. This only works if the damage is smaller than a quarter, and there will still be scarring. When wounds are large, special cells related to muscle cells bridge and contract the wound edges by depositing a random thatch of thin, linear collagen strips. This layer is soon replaced by a layer of aligned, thicker collagen fibers, a spontaneous process called "remodeling." As in a small wound, skin cells may migrate into this emergency scaffolding, but the different scaffold causes skin cells to grow differently—into scar tissue.[8]

The ability of scar tissue to pull together the edges of a wound may save a life, but because it is far less elastic than undamaged skin, scar tissue can also effectively paralyze an otherwise healthy body part. With no sweat glands or hair follicles, the body's ability to regulate heat is also affected, and the patient faces cosmetic disfigurement.

AUTOGRAFT
PROCEDURE FOR
REPLACING A NOSE
Gaspare Tagliocozzi,
Surgeon of Bologna
1597

A flap of skin is lifted up from the patient's arm and sewn onto the face. A special sling holds the patient's arm in position for several weeks while the graft takes hold.

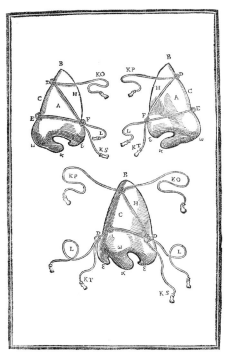

Fig. 68. *De Curtorum Chirurgia.*
Plate XIV

MOLDS FOR SHAPING
GRAFTED SKIN
Gaspare Tagliocozzi,
Surgeon of Bologna
1597

A metal mold is tied around
the head to shape the
grafted skin into a nose.
The skin grows to match the
contours of the mold. Sword
duels made nose and ear
mutilation common during
this period.

PROSTHETICS TO GENETICS

The devastating effects of skin injury have long
motivated research into wound dressing, grafts,
reconstructive surgery, and alternative skins.
Evidence of wound covering has been dated to
1500 B.C.[9] To aid healing and simulate normative
body shape, prosthetic materials abound, many
adapted from the building trades. Materials used
in reconstruction of the nose bridge alone have
historically included rubber, celluloid, iron, copper, platinum, ivory, and
gold. Duck sternum and bone grafts have also been used.[10] Skin repair is
thus an ancient form of augmenting the body with alien materials.

For restoring damaged skin, however, autograft has traditionally
been the most successful treatment, from evidence of its use in sixth-century
India to the present. Autograft uses skin from another part of the patient's
own body. The sixteenth-century surgeon Gaspare Tagliocozzi of Bologna
repaired mutilated noses by sewing skin lifted up from the patient's arm—
still attached to the arm—to the face. After a few weeks, the graft was sev-
ered from from the arm and shaped with a metal mold.[11]

Less arduous forms of autograft are employed today. One type is
called a meshed graft. Using a special meshing tool, harvested skin is perforated with rows of small incisions, allowing the skin to expand over a larger
area. While this technique takes advantage of skin's ability to regenerate
small areas, the healed skin retains a meshed pattern.[12]

Development of a contemporary skin substitute, capable of seamlessly covering larger areas, has depended partly on advances in polymer chemistry. (Polymers are a type of molecule, and the skin's collagen is a type of polymer.) A synthetic polymer called collodion was invented in the 1850s and was used, by the 1860s, to cover and protect wounds. Applied as a liquid, it formed a solid film over the wound site, to be peeled off when the wound healed. Bioabsorbable sutures, common today, were patented in 1963.[13]

Several key developments took place in the late 1970s and early 1980s. First came the observation that applying a certain kind of collagen to a wound blocked its contraction and the formation of scar tissue. Next, researchers found that applying collagen to a wound enabled growth of surviving dermal cells. A third achievement was to grow skin cells on collagen outside of the body and graft the mix sucessfully onto rats. These experiments showed that given the right growth conditions, skin can regenerate.[14]

An optimal scaffold is a fourth key component of viable artificial skin. Both natural and synthetic polymers have been investigated as possible sources. One biotech company developed a way to derive collagen from bovine tendon and to sterilize and purify but not damage it. Another works with pig small intestines discarded from pork production. Another company aimed to construct synthetic polymer micromatrices for artificial skin, using computer-aided design and rapid prototyping machinery like that used in building electronic components.[15]

Bringing together polymers and collagen into artificial skin, investigators sought the following results: full adhesion to a wound, precise moisture flow in and out of the wound, a scaffold structure attractive to dermal cells, flexible strength, a precise biodegradation rate, and acceptability to the body's immune system. "Proof of concept" involved a nonliving, two-layer, temporary skin substitute. The synthetic outer layer prevents infection and regulates fluid loss; an inner layer blocks deposition of scar collagen and provides a scaffold conducive to the growth of migrant skin cells.[16]

Where do the human cells come from to make living skin products? Sometimes the body's own skin cells can be encouraged to grow, but for "off the shelf" artificial skin, a standardized, reproducible source is needed. Some companies producing living skin products collect fibroblasts and ker-

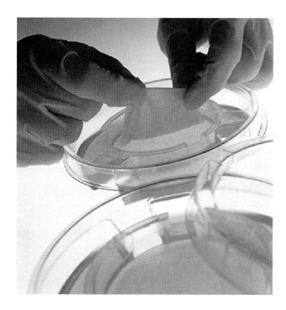

atinocytes from neonatal tissue such as infant human foreskin (leftover from circumcisions). Alternatively, stem cells show great promise for tissue regeneration. Originally identified in newly fertilized eggs, stem cells have been found in bone marrow, brain tissue, and body fat. Stem cells' genetic instructions to differentiate and specialize have yet to be expressed, making it possible to direct their growth. Stem cells in hair follicles have been found to produce skin cells as well as hair.[17]

Another piece of the tissue generation puzzle is the bioreactor, in use by the 1990s. Bioreactors simulate growth conditions in the body, providing a continuous nutrient bath and gentle physical pressure (as from gravity and blood pressure). Some bioreactors bring to mind *Star Trek*'s "Borg maturation chambers," while others appear as simple and disposable as deli containers. One bioreactor is a sealed, sterile plastic cassette. Another is a rotating cylinder (the size of a tomato can) with tubes attached.[18]

In *Sleeper*, Woody Allen is cryogenically preserved and then reheated in aluminum foil; artificial skin also requires special shipping and handling. Some artificial skin products are cryopreserved just prior to shipment, then carefully brought out of stasis for use. TransCyte, for example, is shipped at −36°C; it must be used within forty-eight hours of thawing. Another product, Apligraf, is delivered ready-to-use, and doctors' offices can keep it on hand for up to five days.

The final hurdle for mass production of artificial skin is approval by the U.S. Food and Drug Administration (FDA). Until recently, one factor complicating approval was whether the product was to be considered a device or a pharmaceutical. Artificial skin and other new biotechnologies are neither—and both. In early 2001 the FDA established new regulations affirming a third category called "biologics."[19] The new regulations require producers to follow "Good Tissue Practice" in order to reduce risk of cross-species transmission of dangerous viruses.

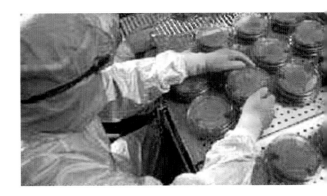

Understanding skin at the chemical, molecular, and genetic levels has enabled this very recent leap from traditional coverings, fillers, and grafts to the professionalization of tissue engineering. *Time* identified it as a job for the future, and *U.S. News and World Report* declared tissue engineering a "hot job track" for 2000.[20]

MASS PRODUCTION
OF LIVING SKIN
COURTESY OF
Organogenesis

SHOPPING

Following these innovations, artificial skin technology has rapidly developed and diversified. There are two basic directions in "skin" products. One approach involves products that contain living skin cells. A second approach uses nonliving material as a temporary barrier, which is applied to a wound to stabilize it and make it receptive to new skin. Then artificial skin is cultured in vitro (or a natural graft is harvested) and applied to the body. A third category of products focuses on wound closure.[21]

Of the products using living skin cells, Apligraf was FDA-approved in 1998. Produced by Organogenesis and marketed by Novartis, Apligraf is a living, two-layer skin product, having both dermis and epidermis. TransCyte and Dermagraft, both by Advanced Tissue Sciences, are formed in bioreactors from a synthetic scaffold seeded with infant foreskin cells. A living, frozen, bi-layer, full-thickness skin substitute is in development from Ortec International.

The second approach encourages the body to grow its own cells. In 1997 the FDA approved a topical gel called Regranex, made by Johnson & Johnson for treatment of diabetic skin ulcers. The active ingredient in Regranex stimulates cell migration to the ulcer site, encouraging growth of new skin.

Dressings temporarily protect a wound while it begins to heal. A layer of pig small intestines called the submucosa has been made into a dressing called OaSIS, by Cook Biotech. Described as "a playground for cell growth" by scientists, the submucosa naturally contains the key elements of collagen, growth factors, and proteins. The submucosa is isolated, washed and sterilized, further stripped down, then freeze-dried into a product resembling parchment paper. North Carolina State University researchers are working on a three-layer dressing formed from chitosan, harvested from animal shells.[22]

Temporary glues and protective finishes that encourage wound closure constitute another area of product development. Anika is a bio-absorbable, implantable membrane designed to prevent post-surgical adhesions. In 2000, Electrosols was designing a spray-on dressing to encourage skin growth following injury. An electric charge in the spray attracts the solution to the skin and causes the tiny polymer fibers to repel each other, arranging themselves in a regular "weave." The electric charge also attracts fibroblasts to the fibers, encouraging skin growth.

BY THE SKIN OF OUR FUTURE

If Woody Allen were frozen today, what would his future be like? If polymers could be made to conduct electricity, artificial nerves could conceivably be developed, or "fast-setting polymers" could be used to fill in a broken bone. Tissue could be engineered to deliver a physiological drug, such as a missing hormone; on this principle, a polymer wafer implant for treatment of brain cancer was introduced in 1997.[23] One team has transplanted egg-laden ovarian tissue into the subdermal muscle in a woman's forearm, where it develops outside of the womb. Reprogenesis is working on a technique for human cells to be harvested, multiplied in the lab, then reimplanted elsewhere in the body to add nondegrading bulk.[24]

If tissue can be made to differentiate into the complex combination of cells making up a working internal organ, livers and hearts could someday be produced for "off-the-shelf" replacement. Or, scaffolds seeded with particular kinds of cells could literally patch up diseased components of organs. Specific tissues have been targeted, such as liver cells grown in the lab and reimplanted. Body parts grown in vitro and sucessfully implanted now include heart valves, thumb bones, intestinal segments, knee cartilage, and even a simulated rib cage.[25] Imagine the human body of the future, its parts continually repaired and replaced by tissue engineers, its outer surface refinished by dermatologists and aesthetic surgeons.

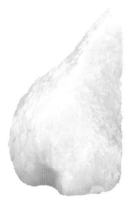

Living cells have been seeded onto a polymer scaffold the shape of a nose; as the cells grow, they replace the polymer with cartilage. An ear is in the works as well, produced in the following way: tissue engineers mold a biodegradable scaffold into the size and shape of an ear, and then seed the scaffold with young cartilage cells. The object is implanted under the skin of a specially bred, hairless mouse. The mouse's body nourishes the ear as the cells grow.[26] The mature ear is surgically removed from the mouse (the mouse survives), and, hypothetically at least, is grafted onto a dictator or anyone else in need of one. In the near future, researchers claim tissue will be custom engineered and transplanted for corrective surgery.

P42

SKIN, the medium of physical contact among living creatures, can be made in a lab and shipped overnight to locations around the world. Cells harvested from one placenta or neonatal foreskin are capable of indefinite growth. Such products challenge our definitions of human life and identity. Skin, containing the full menu of human DNA within a relatively simple organ structure, is among the tissues cryogenically preserved by family members who hope to genetically duplicate their relatives in the cloning facilities of the now-imaginable future. Manufactured skin, which may contain collagen derived from cows and other sources as well as from human skin, is an alien product incorporated into countless bodies. The melding of technology and design into new body surface, new protection, new identity, has come a long way since *Sleeper*. Science, however, has yet to reconstitute a nose flattened by a twenty-first-century steamroller.

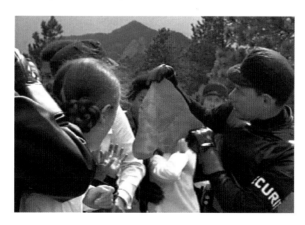

SLEEPER, 1973
DIRECTOR
Woody Allen
WRITERS
Woody Allen and
Marshall Brickman
© United Artists, 1973.

1 Mark C. Taylor, *Hiding* (Chicago: University of Chicago Press, 1997), 12.

2 General information about skin structure and function is from "Skin," *Encyclopedia Britannica Online*. http://search.eb.com.

3 On the science and medicine of blushing, see Atul Gawande, "Crimson Tide," *New Yorker* (February 12, 2001): 50–57.

4 Michael K. Copass, Roy G. Soper, and Mickey S. Eisenberg, *EMT Manual*, 2nd ed. (Philadelphia: W.B. Saunders, 1991), 7.

5 For an analysis of relationships between conceptual and physical differences, see Geoffrey C. Bowker and Susan Leigh Star, *Sorting Things Out: Classification and its Consequences* (Cambridge: MIT Press, 1999).

6 David J. Mooney and Antonios G. Mikos, "Growing New Organs," *Scientific American* 280:4 (April 1999): 63.

7 Ioannis V. Yannas, "Classes of Materials Used in Medicine: Natural Materials," *Biomaterials Science: An Introduction to Materials in Medicine* (San Diego: Academic Press, 1996), 85.

8 Frederick H. Silver, *Biomaterials, Medical Devices and Tissue Engineering: An Integrated Approach* (London: Chapman & Hall, 1994), 64–65.

9 Ioannis V. Yannas, "Artificial Skin and Dermal Equivalents," *Biomedical Engineering Handbook*, Joseph D. Bronzino, ed. (Boca Raton, Fla.: CRC, 1995), 2026.

10 Sander L. Gilman, *Making the Body Beautiful: A Cultural History of Aesthetic Surgery* (Princeton: Princeton University Press, 1999), 57.

11 Martha Teach Gnudi and Jerome Pierce Webster, *The Life and Times of Gaspare Tagliacozzi, Surgeon of Bologna, 1545–1599* (Milan: Ulrico Hoepli, 1965).

12 Yannas, "Artificial Skin and Dermal Equivalents," 2027.

13 David J. Tennenbaum, "People and Polymers," *Beyond Discovery: The Path from Research to Human Benefit* (Washington, D.C.: National Academy of Sciences, 2001). http://www4.nas.edu/beyond/beyonddiscovery.nsf/web/polymers?OpenDocument.

14 Key developments are reviewed in Frederick H. Silver and George Pins, "Cell Growth on Collagen: A Review of Tissue Engineering Using Scaffolds Containing Extracellular Matrix," *Journal of Long Time Effects of Medical Implants* 2:1 (1992): 67–80.

15 Nancy Parenteau, "The Organogenesis Story," *Scientific American* 280:4 (April 1999): 83; E. Bell, H. P. Ehrlich, D. J. Buttle, et al., "Living Tissue Formed in Vitro and Accepted as Skin-Equivalent Tissue of Full Thickness," *Science* 211: 1052–54; Diane Martindale, "Scar No More," *Scientific American* (July 2000): http://www.sciam.com/2000/0700issue/0700techbus1.html; Gale Morrison, "Advances in the Skin Trade," *Mechanical Engineering*, 40–43.

16 Yannas, "Artifical Skin and Dermal Equivalents," 2028–34.

17 Nichalas Wade, "Hair Follicles Identified as Probable Home of Skin's Stem Cells," *New York Times* (August 18, 2000): A23; and Denise Grady, "Fat is Good Source of Stem Cells, a Study Says," *New York Times* (April 10, 2001): A15.

18 Robert S. Langer and Joseph P. Vacanti, "Tissue Engineering: The Challenges Ahead," *Scientific American* 280:4 (April 1999): 86.

19 For details see Center for Biologics Evaluation and Research, http://www.fda.gov/cber/.

20 "Visions of the 21st Century: Our Work, Our World," *Time.com* (May 1, 2000): http://www.time.com/time/reports/v21/work/mag_ten_hottest_jobs.html; and *U.S. News and World Report* (November 1, 1999): http://www.usnews.com/usnews/issue/991101/nycu/core20.htm.

21 These products are described in "Wound Care Products—Corporate Developments," *Medical and Healthcare Marketplace Guide* (Philadelphia: Dorlands Directories, 1998), vol. I.

22 Martindale, "Scar No More."

23 Gerald Parkinson, "Melding Medicine with Engineering," *Chemical Engineering* (May 1998): 28–29.

24 Lila Gutterman, "An Armful of Eggs: Ovarian Transplants Could Restore Lost Fertility," *Chronicle of Higher Education* (January 26, 2001): A19.

25 Catherine Arnst and John Carey, "Biotech Bodies" *Business Week* (July 27, 1998): http://www.businessweek.com/1998/30/coverstory.htm.

26 "The Bionic Body: The Body Shop," *Scientific American Frontiers*, http://www. pbs.org/saf/1107/features/body.htm

EYEBEAM MUSEUM/ATELIER
COMPETITION, 2001
Digital rendering
DESIGNER Greg Lynn, b. 1964
Greg Lynn FORM, Los Angeles

This competition entry for a new museum of art and technology in New York City uses the undulating skin of the building as a vast screen for electronic imagery. With this proposal, architect Greg Lynn asserts that the surface of the building is more valuable than its interior. The tower has become a medium in itself, another channel for broadcast. The building's skin drapes into deep folds at its base, creating spatial pockets that act as portals to the museum.

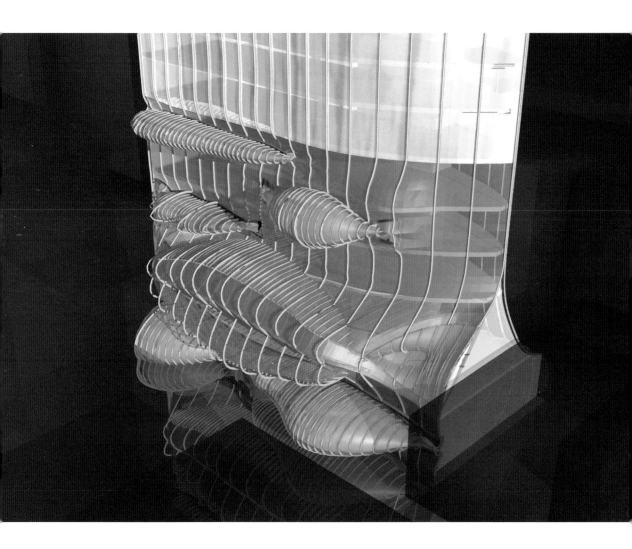

ALICIA IMPERIALE

digital
skins

THE ARCHITECTURE OF SURFACE

QUESTIONS REGARDING SKIN are profound, not superficial. Where are its boundaries? What is its status? Is it surface or depth or both? Skin is the space of flux, of oscillating conditions. When Paul Valéry once noted, ironically, that "the skin is the deepest," he drew attention to skin as a surface of maximum interface and intensity. The use of body images and metaphors to discuss cultural phenomena have influenced discussions of art, architecture, and design over the past decade. In broad cultural terms, there has been a movement away from dialectical relationships, from the opposition between surface and depth, in favor of an awareness of the oscillating movement from one into the other. Smooth exchange, flow, continuous surface, skin, membranes, bubbles—these concepts are ever-present in contemporary culture, from animation to economics. They signal a paradigm shift in the relationship between humans and technology. As the human becomes increasingly technological, the distinction between the natural and the made have blurred. The design tools used in film, architecture, and product design have amplified and accelerated our ability to represent the collapse of nature into technology. Digital 3d modeling software uses algorithmic formulas to generate and change soft, curved form in an auto-catalytic system resembling genetic mutation.

Portions of this text have been adapted from Imperiale's *New Flatness: Surface Tension in Digital Architecture* (Basel: Birkhauser Publishers, 2000).

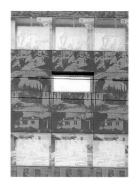

CONTEMPORARY ARCHITECTS are confronting the focus on surface and skin in today's culture and technology. In the early twentieth century, modernists sought to simultaneously convey the tension between deep space and surface, often through the use of glass and other transparent surfaces. This set up a dialectical division between the interior and exterior of a building.[1]

Today, some architects compress allusions to the depth of the interior into the surface or skin of a building. Jacques Herzog and Pierre de Meuron address shells, layers, and wraps in their buildings. Exterior skins are built up through layers of veiling, or are inscribed with figurative imagery, invoking what might lie behind the surface. The Eberswalde Technical School Library, in Eberswalde, Germany, has images pressed into the building's concrete surface and silkscreened onto the glass windows. What remains is a "tattooed concrete skin."[2] While each frame is a single image, the images are bound into repetitive ribbons that encircle the building, unifying the whole. The use of the continuous imagery on both the glass and the concrete belies the inherent nature of each material: the glass becomes semi-opaque while the concrete attains a shimmering lightness.

The living skin varies dramatically as it adapts to the exigencies of the body—thick where the skeleton needs some padding to soften contact, hardened in response to friction. If eyelids were completely opaque, one would lose a critical mechanism in the waking process. The skin of architecture can also be differentiated. Kamiel Klaasse of NL Architects describes the project WOS 8, an electrical cooling station, as a simple sculptural object. The entire surface is coated with seamless polyurethane, creating a protective enclosure for an internal mechanism. The skin helps to reduce heat and noise emissions. The sides of the volume are also varied; there is a climbing wall, a bird wall, a basketball wall, and so on. Klaasse describes the building as "a public square wrapped around a machine." He sculpted the initial form by hand and used advanced 3d modeling software to facilitate the analysis and manufacturing of the complex form.[3]

1 On the depthlessness of surface, see Fredric Jameson, *Postmodernism, or, The Cultural Logic of Late Capitalism* (Raleigh-Durham, N.C.: Duke University Press, 1991). On biomorphism in contemporary art and design, see Mark Dery, "Exquisite Corpses" *Bookforum* (summer 2001): 5–6.
2 Sarah Amelar, "Two Herzog & de Meuron Projects Reveal Deep Skin," *Architectural Record* (August 1999): 82–91.
3 Kamiel Klaasse, telephone interview with the author, 28 June 2001.

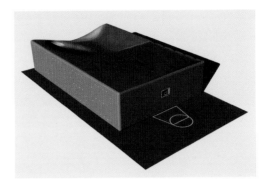

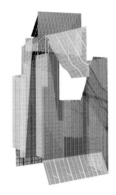

Le Corbusier used elements such as the roof terrace and the brise-soleil to adapt the skins of his buildings to different climates. Such additions were considered a part of the exterior structure of the building. In the recent Village Fashion Center, in Seoul, Korea by Morphosis and in the Recyclable, Portable Skyscraper by FTL Happold, external elements such as sun-shading louvers are not considered one with the skin's structure in a modernist sense. These projects peel away or build up their skins as a series of differentiated masks and layers. There is no definite exterior or interior but a gradual movement from outside to inside through an ensemble of inflected parts.

A living body may be imagined as a continuous surface from inside to out, but there are limits to the actual representation of that continuity.[4] Medical technology has continually sought to uncover the unseen, the unknown, that hides behind a body's surface. Through time this imaging has moved from the surface of the body to probing its depths. While photographic methods have an analog relationship to the body, newer forms of imaging translate information from non-invasive probings into universal digital binary code. Density of bone, tissue, neural impulses, blood flow—all these are registered in a precise series of 0s and 1s.

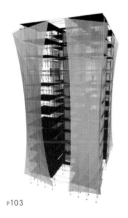

Digital technologies that were once used to image an existing opaque object have been appropriated by designers to project new bodies, new spaces, new architectures. Forms designed within the space of the

---

4 The layering and folding of matter that forms all bodies is discussed in Gilles Deleuze, *The Fold: Leibniz and the Baroque* (Minnesota: University of Minnesota Press, 1993), and Bernard Cache, *Earth Moves: The Furnishing of Territories* (Cambridge: MIT Press, 1995). On the fold in architecture, see Greg Lynn, ed., "Folding in Architecture," *Architectural Design* (London: Academy Editions, 1993).

computer are analogous to bodies moving in time. The area of digital technology that has had a critical impact on design and architecture is the realm of NURBS-based (Non-Uniform Rational Bézier Spline) 3d modeling programs such as Alias, Catia, Rhinoceros, Pro/Engineer, and Maya, which allow designers to create new "bodies" and to work with complex curvatures in real time.[5]

NURBS-based programs contrast with other extensively used specific software programs such as AutoCad that rely on Cartesian forms. While a CAD/CAM (computer-aided design and manufacturing) program such as AutoCad is versatile, it does not encourage design with fluid curvatures. This kind of program is based on locators for every point, line, plane, or curve in the Cartesian X, Y, and Z coordinate system. In contrast, programs based on NURB splines and curves use algorithmic formulas to allow lines and surfaces to be adjusted and recalculated continuously.

A curved surface is created by a series of these splines, and the curved surface is constantly recalculated in relation to such points. New surfaces are embedded and developed in relation to the existing surface. Similarly, the geometry itself is defined relative to the surface. If you change scale in a part of the surface, the entire surface is rescaled, recalculated. NURBS programs are based on an inherently dynamic system: surfaces and objects are developed in a shifting relation to a surface. Rather than conceiving of form as a static condition, the new 3d modeling software programs allow the designer to work on a form that is constantly evolving, smoothly registering the continuously changing algorithmic parameters in 3d topological surfaces before the designer's eye and through the designer's intervention.[6]

---

5 See Greg Lynn, *Animate Form* (New York: Princeton Architectural Press, 1999); and Gerald Farin, *NURBS Curves and Surfaces from Projective Geometry to Practical Use* (Wellesley, MA: A. K. Peters, 1995). This section is also informed by Cory Clarke, interview with the author.
6 Topology is the study of the behavior of a surface structure under deformation.

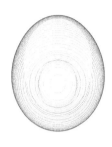

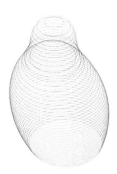

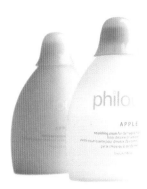

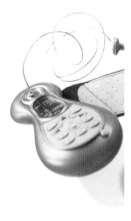

AVO PHONE, 2000
Memory Elastomer, ABS, and
electronic components
DESIGNERS Yves Béhar and
Joshua Morenstein
frogdesign, Sunnyvale,
California
MATERIALS ADVISOR
Angelita Tadeo
PHOTOGRAPHY Mark Serr

Product designers have used these technologies for over a decade; application of various advanced 3d modeling software programs has had a liberating effect on the design process, in the design and visualization and the prototyping and manufacturing phases. Yves Béhar's plastic Philou bottle is conceived as the intersection of two perfect egg-shapes. The inherent asymmetries in the geometry of the egg are used to poignant effect, with the bottle leaning slightly to the side, seemingly in motion, and ripe with life. Although Béhar's designs begin with hand sketches, these intuitions are then developed in the program Alias, which allows him to understand the form with a mathematical exactitude and to manufacture the product directly from a digital file.

Béhar uses the more robust program Pro/E for products that necessitate integration among complex surface and mechanical elements. His design for Avo, a mobile telephone, demanded coordination between the interior components and their outer covering. As different portions of the design evolved, each change was automatically carried through to all other aspects of the product, allowing a seamless integration between the skin and the interior mechanism of the product. It is this aspect of parametric design that brings to mind prior discussions of the continuity of skin.[7]

---

7 Yves Béhar, telephone interview with the author, 29 June 2001.

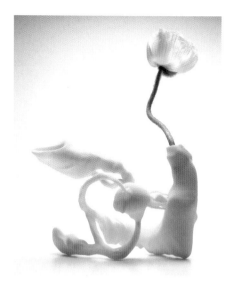

What's in a sneeze? Using a powerful 3d digital scanner, designer Marcel Wanders makes the invisible visible. In his Airborne Snotty Vase series, he has captured the form of molecular compounds from the airborne sneezes of people suffering from a variety of ailments (influenza, ozaena, pollinosis, sinusitis, coryza). The sneezes were captured by a 3d particle scanner, and the microscopic components were then selected and enlarged 100 times. Imported into a 3d modeling program, the exterior forms of the components were maintained, while the interiors were hollowed out. This information was then sent to a rapid prototyping machine in order to make the studies for the vases. Digital tools have allowed Wanders not only to work with form that is beyond the grasp of human vision, but to work with forms of an extreme complexity from the design phase to production.[8]

Three-dimensional modeling software is relatively new for architecture. Many of the 3d software programs being used by architects were not originally developed for architectural practice. CAD/CAM systems, CNC milling systems, Alias, Maya—these tools were developed for the manufacturing of consumer products, from automobiles and toothbrushes to airplanes and special effects for film. Architects are now using these technologies to design and manufacture architectural elements, which are then brought together to produce a sinuous, inflected architecture of variation.

[8] Marcel Wanders with the author, 2 July 2001.

Greg Lynn addresses the design of networked surfaces in his Embryonic House project, a prototype for prefabricated housing that consists of a skin composed of more than 3,000 individual panels. Because the system is networked, a change in any component of the system is registered in other parts of the skin. The surfaces are designed with 3d modeling software to attain a fluid form. Study models and the full-scale panels are manufactured utilizing computer-controlled milling and cutting machinery with the same digital data. This coordinated design and manufacturing system has the advantage of generating maximum differentiation in the simple configuration of the surface, as a real skin would deform and change in a living body. This is also evident in his recent proposal for the Eyebeam competition (a museum and atelier for video and electronic art), in which the internal organs push to the surface of the building's skin.

Sulan Kolatan and William Mac Donald examine the relationship of consumer objects and the potential for hybridization with building. Cut an athletic shoe in half, Kolatan and Mac Donald suggest, and you find various cavities, layers, and bladders. The shoe, through the layering of surfaces, employs flexible, responsive materials that mediate between itself and the body as well as the ground. An analysis of the shoe raises many new ideas of surface layering—they may be fused, sewn, constructed from silicone—and these may be used to influence materiality and construction in architecture.

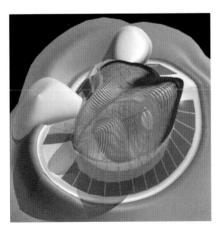

EMBRYONIC HOUSE
Digital rendering
DESIGNER Greg Lynn, b. 1964
Greg Lynn FORM, Los Angeles

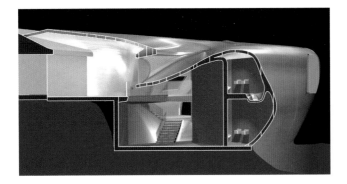

Surface and sectional conditions of Kolatan and Mac Donald's Raybould House suggest the bladders, skins, and surfaces evident in the shoe. There is, of course, a scalar and material shift (aluminum, stretched across ribs) in the house. Kolatan and Mac Donald have used the animation software Maya to mediate between architecture and landscape. Although the Raybould project is static, its openness and curvature evoke the shoe's ability to negotiate between body and environment.

Architects have appropriated many terms and concepts from philosopher Gilles Deleuze's work *The Fold*: affiliation, smooth and striated space, folding, and pliancy. The incorporation of these terms, which Deleuze developed to describe baroque aesthetics and thought, into architectural practice has led to significant changes in how buildings are thought of in relation to the environment. Deleuzean thought has promoted smoother transitions and interactive exchanges across surfaces through serendipitous, temporary links that exist within buildings and sites. The fold is ambiguous, being figure and nonfigure, organization and nonorganization. As a formal metaphor, the fold has appealed to architects who seek to move past highly figured and readily identified form to an architecture that is rather formless.

The design of smooth form has been facilitated by architects' access to time-based NURBS modeling software such as Alias and Maya. In this sense, the use of digital technologies has had a liberating effect on architectural form. Architects can design organic, bodylike architectures that register the infinite variations and mutations from their evolutionary growth stage in built form. These sinuous curvatures and warped surfaces wrap around the inhabitant like a second skin. The elision between the inhabitant and the architecture, between the object and the user, the landscape and building, is symptomatic of our time.

WHEN USING NURBS-BASED SOFTWARE, one creates an object by connecting one surface to another. The surface, skin, and interface of architecture is emphasized, instigating a more technical, performative, programmatic, and environmental way of thinking, one that has its roots in the language of building. Yet there is a superfluous character of interior space that results from placing so much emphasis on the design of the architectural skin and its supporting structure. While the design of a sinuous architecture theoretically seeks to smooth distinctions between the exterior and interior, this division is actually heightened. There is the risk of the architectural interior becoming merely the leftover space of a highly articulated bloblike exterior. Architectural theorist Anthony Vidler sees this division as consistent with the severing of the inside and the outside of built form as suggested by Deleuze.[9] Yet in the examples of baroque architecture discussed by Deleuze, there is a strong contrast between the interior and exterior that makes the architecture dynamic. In much contemporary architecture, that division melts away.

The desire to make a smooth architecture ties into a broader cultural discussion. We are living in a moment when rounded contours, malleable materials, and skinlike finishes grace the smooth bodies and objects we touch daily. Three-dimensioanl digital modeling software plays a large role in this discussion. It is remarkable that 3d modeling applications can be used to design a handheld consumer object or an urban-scale intervention. This sliding scale in the digital continuum equalizes previously distinct cultural artifacts. What results is a strange fetishism of the consumer object, an emphasis on the intimate interface between technology and the living body. It is the moment where the terror of the technological is softened through smooth contours between our hands and the objects we use and the architectures and urban surfaces that surround us.

9 Anthony Vidler, "Skin and Bones: Folded Forms from Leibniz to Lynn," in *Warped Space: Art, Architecture, and Anxiety in Modern Culture* (Cambridge: MIT Press, 2000), 230.

beauty,
horror
+
biotechnology

SKIN is the body part most easily altered by human beings, from circumcision and scarification to cosmetics and hair removal. Popular demand for aesthetic surgery and dermatology soared in the 1990s. At the same time, tissue engineers were learning to manufacture living skin in laboratories. Science fiction explores the extreme possibilities of human/machine hybrids in the figure of the cyborg, a living creature with electromechanical body parts. We are already cyborgs, however, equipped with cell phones, pacemakers, hearing aids, and other prosthetics.

Designers have confronted the medical and mechanical transformation of the human body with horror as well as fascination. The beauty of bodies and objects is submerged in the realm of the artificial, from synthetic materials to digitally manipulated surfaces. The walls of buildings bend, morph, and glow. Eroticism comes clothed in latex, as an aesthetic of hygiene—kinky and clean— envelops the surfaces we touch.

LIPS AND HAIR, 1999

Photograph

PHOTOGRAPHY Elinor Carucci, b. 1971

COURTESY OF Ricco/Maresca Gallery, New York

Carucci's photographs explore the intimate relations
between the body and the routine technologies of
beauty and fashion, from lipstick to zippers.

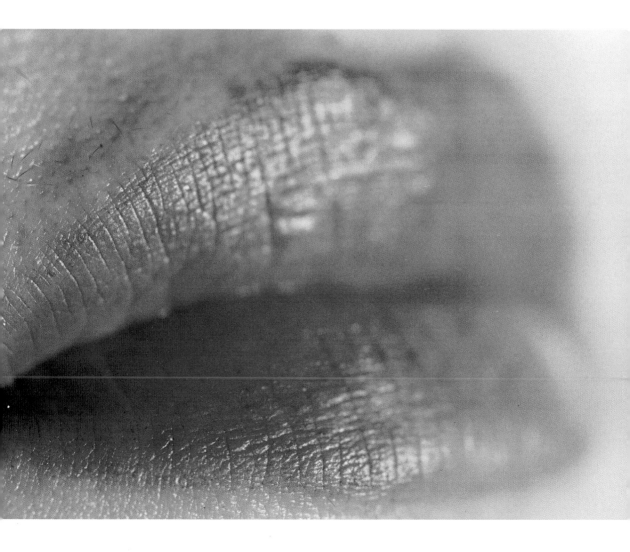

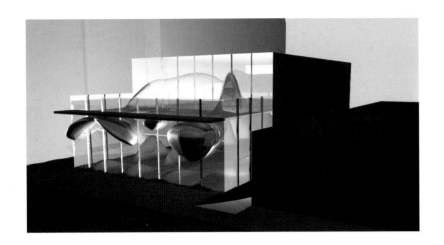

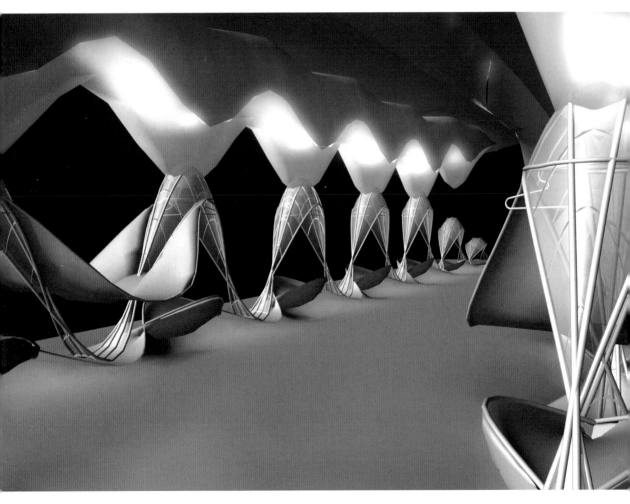

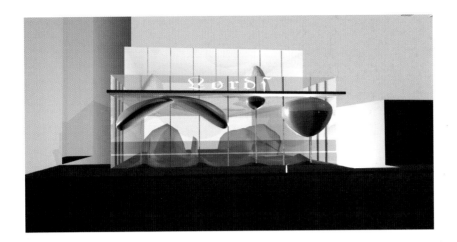

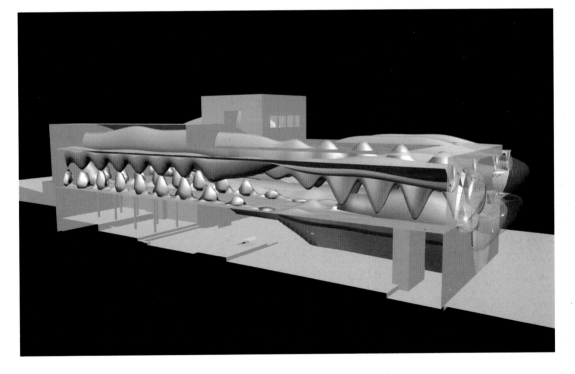

LORD'S ON SUNSET, LOS ANGELES
2001
Digital renderings
DESIGNER Greg Lynn, b. 1964
Greg Lynn FORM, Los Angeles

Lord's is a retail store purveying high-end "rock star" clothing. The exterior of the store's new location on Sunset Boulevard will consist of a glazed box penetrated by a series of folded curves that run from the front to the back of the building. Display spaces ("gems") are created where the folded forms penetrate the front and rear facades. The interior spaces fold and turn, vertically connecting the three levels of the building. An advanced computer-controlled manufacturing system will be used to economically fabricate the folded interior skins, while a more conventional glazing system will complete the exterior box.

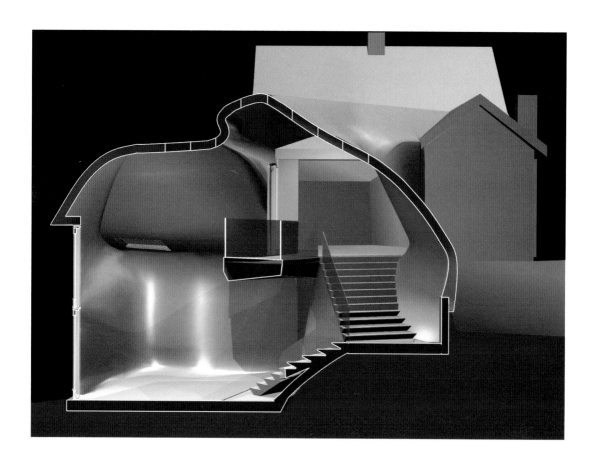

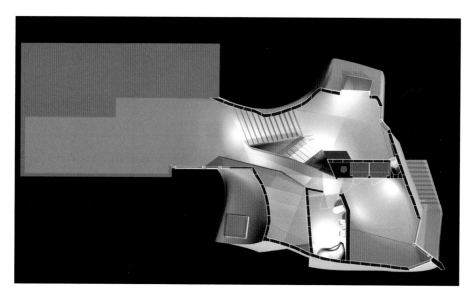

RAYBOULD HOUSE AND GARDEN
FAIRFIELD COUNTY, CONNECTICUT
1997
Digital renderings
DESIGNERS   Sulan Kolatan, b. 1958
William Mac Donald, b. 1956
Kolatan/Mac Donald Studios, New York

Architects Sulan Kolatan and William Mac Donald designed this extension for an existing house as a flowing object grafted onto the landscape. Just as living skin wraps continuously from the surface of the body into the cavities of the nose and ear, the skin of this building flows into the interior spaces. The skeleton of the building consists of plywood ribs cut with a computer-driven milling machine, enabling the construction of the building's complex curves.

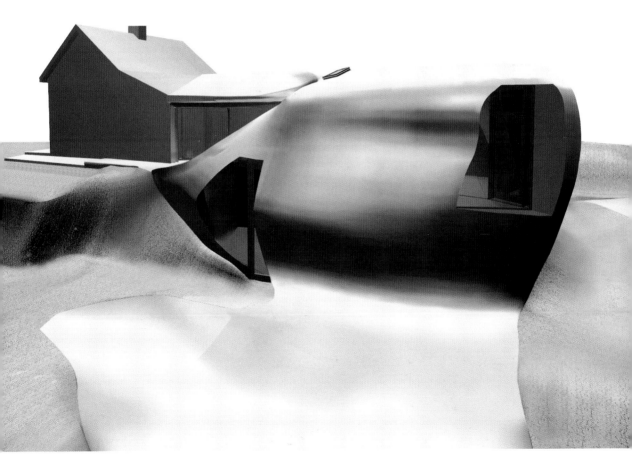

WOS 8, UTRECHT, 1997–98

Heat transfer station

Digital rendering and photographs

DESIGNERS NL Architects, Netherlands, in cooperation with
ir. Djin Sie (Bureau Nieuwbouw Centrales UNA N.V.)

PROJECT ARCHITECTS Pieter Bannenberg, Walter van Dijk, Mark Linnemann,
Kamiel Klaasse

COLLABORATORS Quirijn Calis, Florian Idenburg, Eliana Mello, Michel Schreinemachers,
Ruud Visser

CLIENT Energieproduktiebedrijf (energy production company) UNA N.V.,
Bureau Nieuwbouw Centrales, Utrecht

CONTRACTOR Van Zoelen B.V.

ENGINEER DHV AIB BV

WOS 8 is a heat transfer station. A large power plant about a kilometer away is cooled with water that contains enough energy to supply 11,000 dwellings with heat and warm water. WOS 8 is the node where the loop from the power plant transfers its energy. Before it was built, this energy was dumped as waste heat into the Amsterdam-Rhine canal. The footprint of the building exactly equals the available plot—architecture is reduced to a skin-deep zone.

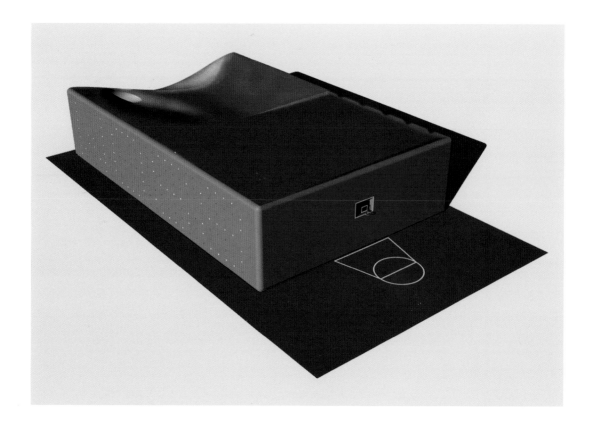

"The building is a public square wrapped around a machine." —NL Architects

"Our client basically asked us to design a skin. We took this seriously. Up until the present most architecture explicitly defines, and is defined by, top, front, and bottom. Different materials fulfill different functions: roof tiles on the roof, bricks for the facade, concrete for walls and floors, etc. Today, there is a new type of wrap available. A membrane of polyurethane enables architecture to become seamless. The material was originally developed for parking roofs: strong, flexible, waterproof, durable, attractive, and chemically inert (no pollution of earth and ground water). It is easily applicable by spray gun or paint roller. Building parts that might refer to scale or size, like doors, disappear." —NL Architects

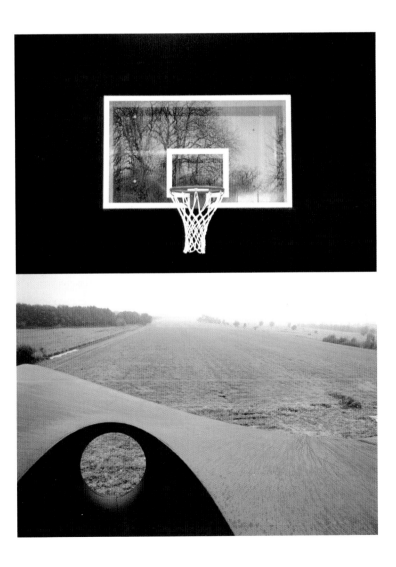

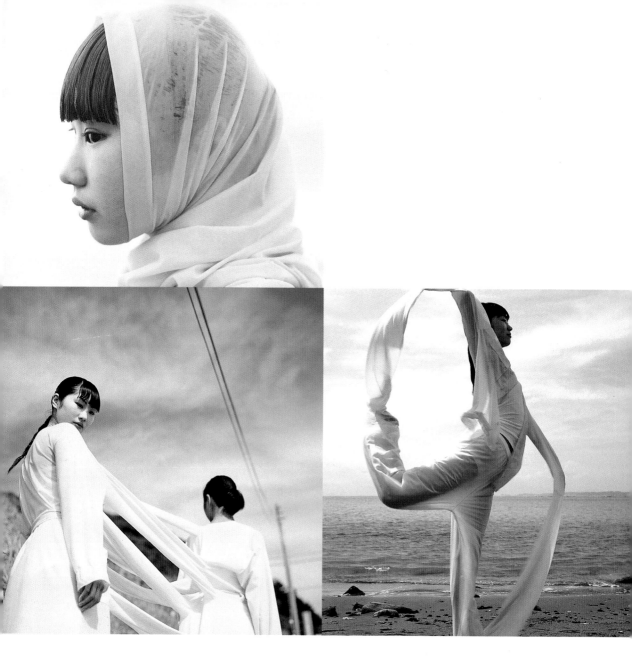

FRESH, 1998–2000
Latex garments

DESIGNER Matthieu Manche, b. 1969
MANUFACTURER Fresh, Japan
PHOTOGRAPHY Kenshu Shintsubo
HAIR + MAKEUP Kenji Ishida (Kiki)
STYLING Aomi
MODEL Shiho Ochiai

When used to manufacture condoms or gloves, latex closely follows the contours of the human body. Artist and designer Matthieu Manche uses latex to suggest, instead, an elaboration and overflowing of the body. Pouches and containers for new growths appear across the surfaces of his clothing, while tubes of latex link body parts and entire bodies into new configurations.

"Latex is similar to the skin, but it
is extremely artificial. I try to unsettle
people's expectations about skin."
—Matthieu Manche

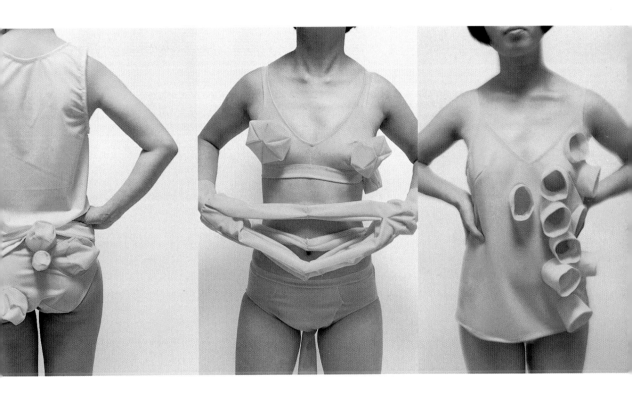

FRESH, 1998–2000
Latex garments
DESIGNER Matthieu Manche
MANUFACTURER Fresh, Japan
PHOTOGRAPHY Matthieu Manche

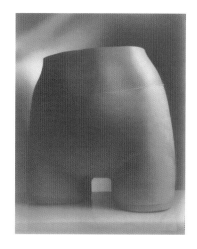

"Sensate aims to bridge the gap between the medical devices we have to protect ourselves and the erotic paraphernalia we use to express and enjoy ourselves."
—Tonita Abeyta

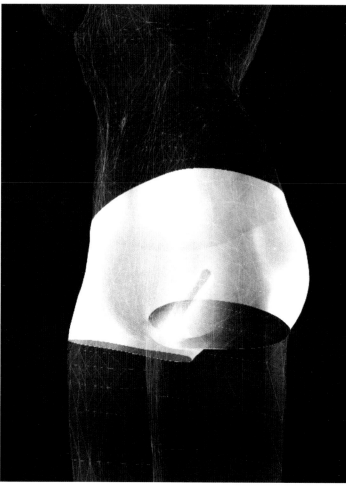

SENSATE, 2000–2001

Protoype, latex panty with integrated condom

Digital rendering and photographs

DESIGNER Tonita Abeyta, b. 1965

MANUFACTURER (PROTOTYPE)

California Medical Innovations, U.S.A.

PHOTOGRAPHY Jeffrey Newbury

ALIAS RENDERING Fooey Studios

Tonita Abeyta is designing a full line of latex garments, with and without built-in male or female condoms. The female condom rendered at left will not slip out of place while in use and does not require an outer ring to stay in place. Some pieces in the Sensate line are pure fashion (such as tops, gloves, and stockings). They coordinate with the wearable condoms for a complete "look." Abeyta believes that a sense of fun and comfort will help achieve the larger goal of integrating safer sexual practices into the public consciousness. The garments are made by dipping a mold (called a mandrel, top left) into liquid latex. A single mold can be used to create garments with different cuts, such as bikini and brief.

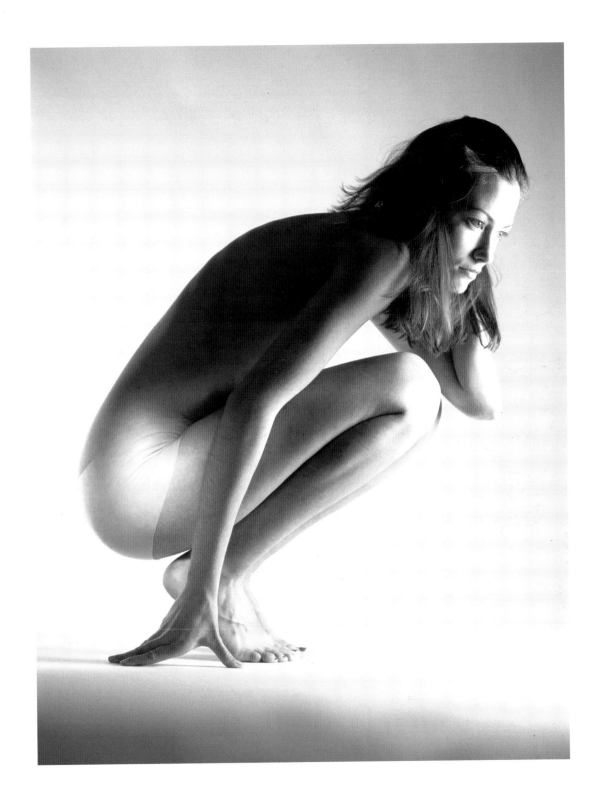

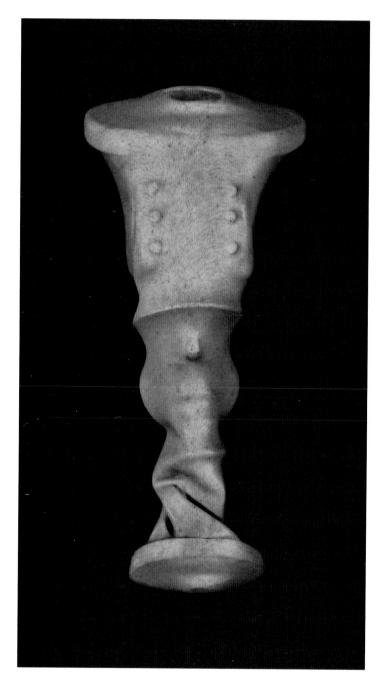

CHIMERA NO. 5 (LEFT)
CHIMERA NO. 8 (RIGHT)
Photographs, 1998
PHOTOGRAPHY
Anthony Aziz, b. 1961
Sammy Cucher, b. 1958
Aziz + Cucher, New York
COURTESY OF
Henry Urbach Architecture,
New York

Aziz + Cucher create digitally
modified photographs of
objects and space covered in
skin. Here, a latex tube stuffed
with electronics components is
the substrate.

"We experience the new biotechnological reality as both something comforting and disconcerting....
In the mid to late 1980s, in relation to AIDS, the abjection of the body was its 'truth'; one couldn't understand the body in any other way because all we knew was illness and death. Now living with AIDS as an active body with a future is my reality."
—Sammy Cucher

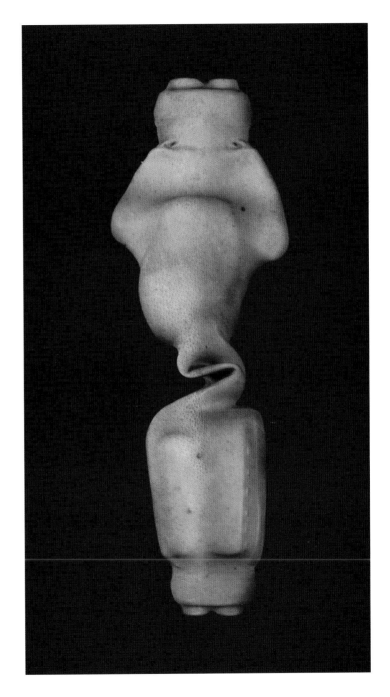

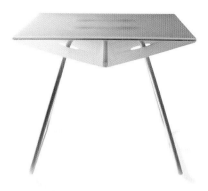

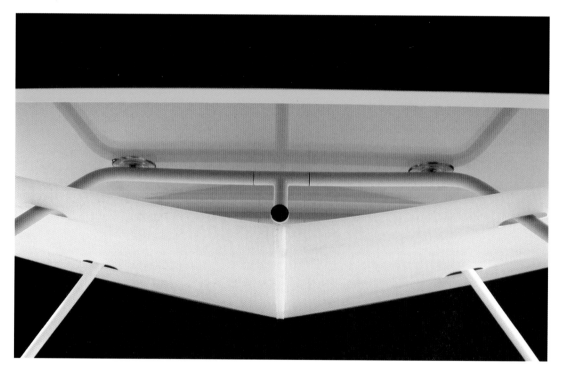

DB-1 AND DB-2, 2001
Table, laminated glass and acrylic,
translucent PVC skin, powder-
coated steel, rubber, nylon glides

DESIGNERS   Dakota Jackson, b. 1949
            Marissa Brown, b. 1968
MANUFACTURER   Dakota Jackson Inc., New York
PHOTOGRAPHY   Dakota Jackson

A soft, translucent skin wraps around a
skeleton of rigid materials. Like a slice through
a living creature, the edge view of the table
reveals the layering and interpenetration of
diverse materials.

KOKON DOUBLE CHAIR, 1999
PVC coating, existing wooden chairs
DESIGNER   Jurgen Bey, b. 1965
Droog Design Collection
PHOTOGRAPHY   Bob Goedewaagen

Jurgen Bey's Kokon series encloses traditional wooden furnishings inside a tight wrapping of PVC, often binding two or more objects into a new whole. The familiar, humanly scaled limbs of the found objects press through the grossly artificial exterior. The "natural" object is at once concealed and objectified within its plastic cocoon. Bey employs the "spiderweb" technique, which is used in aircraft construction to cover open parts.

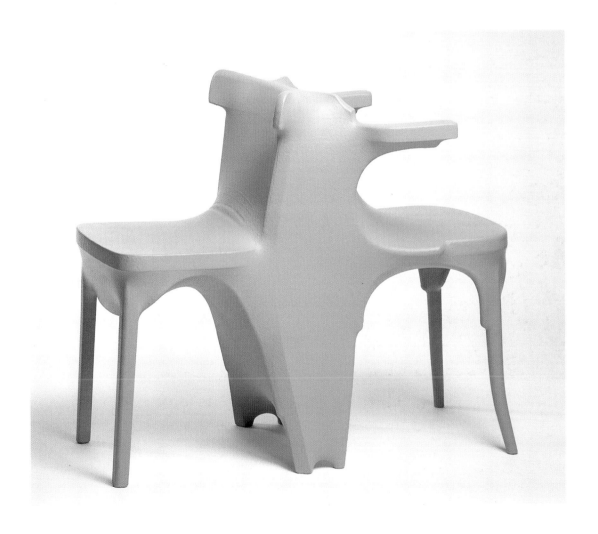

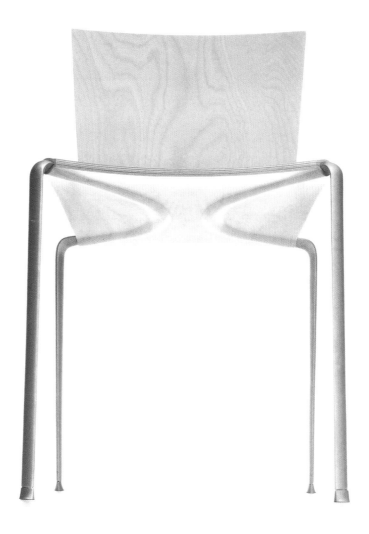

TAINO CHAIR, 2000
Beech, aluminum
DESIGNER Jakob Gebert, b. 1965
MANUFACTURER Vitra, Germany
PHOTOGRAPHY Hans Hansen

The Taino chair expands on the modernist fascination with molded plywood furniture. Producing such chairs has been difficult because of complications in the joining of wood and metal. Here, the metal legs of the chair pass between layers of wood, which are molded around them. Thus the metal does does not have to be fastened to the wood with separate hardware, but is held in place by the skin. The structure shows through the base like bones or veins.

"Red Hot Nude is an exploration of biomorphic form in synthetic materials. I was interested in reskinning the form with a transparent material, therefore exposing the 'innards' or structure."
—Elizabeth Paige Smith

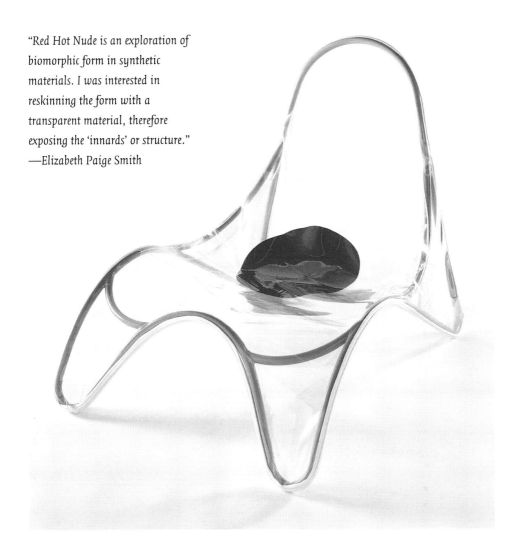

RED HOT NUDE, 2001

Chair, UV vinyl, powder-coated stainless steel frame, zipper

DESIGNER Elizabeth Paige Smith, b. 1968

PHOTOGRAPHY Lynn Campbell

The metal frame of Elizabeth Paige Smith's Red Hot Nude chair is sandwiched between two layers of vinyl, which are attached together with a continuous zipper along the perimeter of the frame. The red dot—the erotic hot spot at the center of the nude—is a flat piece of material adhered to the inside bottom layer of the vinyl.

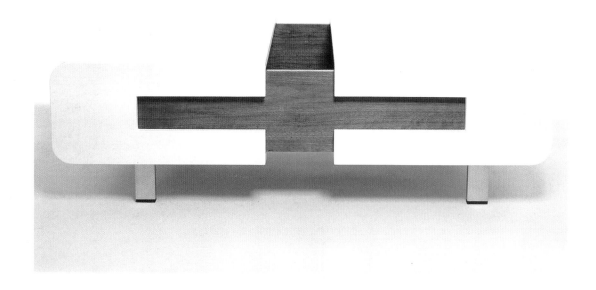

FOUR FORTY, 2000
Table, walnut, steel, laquered wood
DESIGNER   Michael Solis, b. 1969
MANUFACTURER   Dune, New York
PHOTOGRAPHY   Nick Vaccaro

The pristine white shell of this coffee table pulls apart to reveal an interior drawer, designed to hold up to 440 CDs. Dune's Urburbia line of furniture was conceived to maximize space in city dwellings.

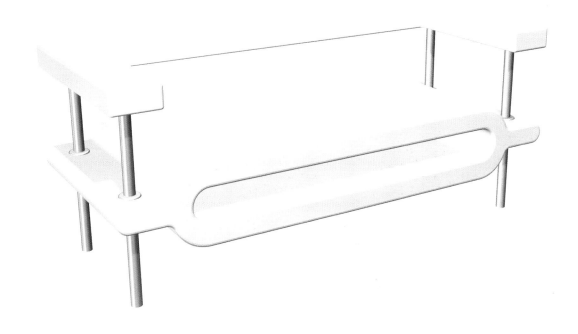

MAGAZINE SOFA, 1997

Vinyl, steel

DESIGNER Michael Young, b. 1966

M. Y. Studio, London

MANUFACTURER Twentytwentyone, London

The smooth upholstered volume of the Magazine couch wraps around an interior cavity, designed for holding magazines or newspapers. The skin is a continuous covering for interior and exterior forms and spaces.

MAGNET, 1998

Cabinet prototype, magnetic rubber, steel

DESIGNER Jan Melis, b. 1966

To open this cabinet, which has a magnetized
rubber door, the user peels back the skin.
A surface one expects to be hard proves to be
soft and flexible.

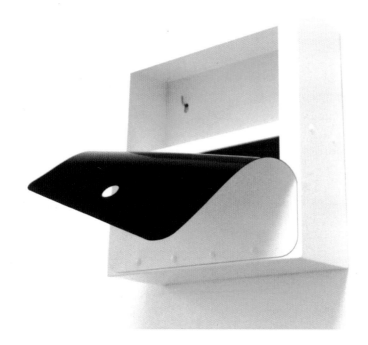

LATEX CUPBOARD, 1999

Steel, wood, latex

DESIGNER Chris Slutter, b. 1962

MANUFACTURER DMD, Netherlands

Droog Design Collection

PHOTOGRAPHY Marsel Loermans

This cabinet has a latex-covered door.
When objects are placed inside, they press
against the cabinet's outer membrane.

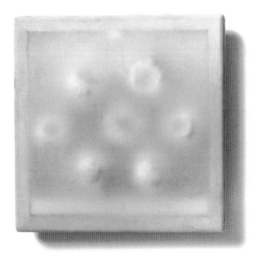
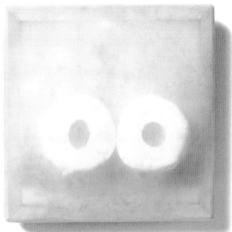

PUSHED WASHBASIN 1

1996

Soft polyurethane

DESIGNER

Hella Jongerius, b. 1963

MANUFACTURER

Hella Jongerius, Netherlands

Droog Design Collection

PHOTOGRAPHY

Bob Goedewaagen

This sink by Hella Jongerius, photographed in her own studio, is made from soft resin. The hard, opaque surface of the traditional bathroom becomes yielding and translucent.

BATHROOM MAT, 1993

Soft polyurethane

DESIGNER

Hella Jongerius

MANUFACTURER

DMD, Netherlands

Droog Design Collection

PHOTOGRAPHY

Dan Meyers

Jongerius's bathroom mat is bubbled with soft, domed protrusions. Like drops of water captured in a solid state, the bubbles massage the feet within the typically hard, cold space of the bathroom.

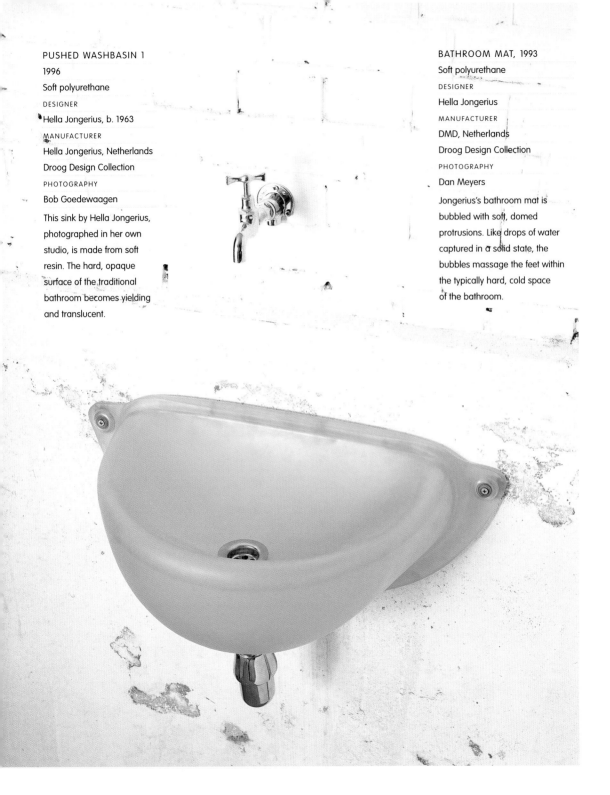

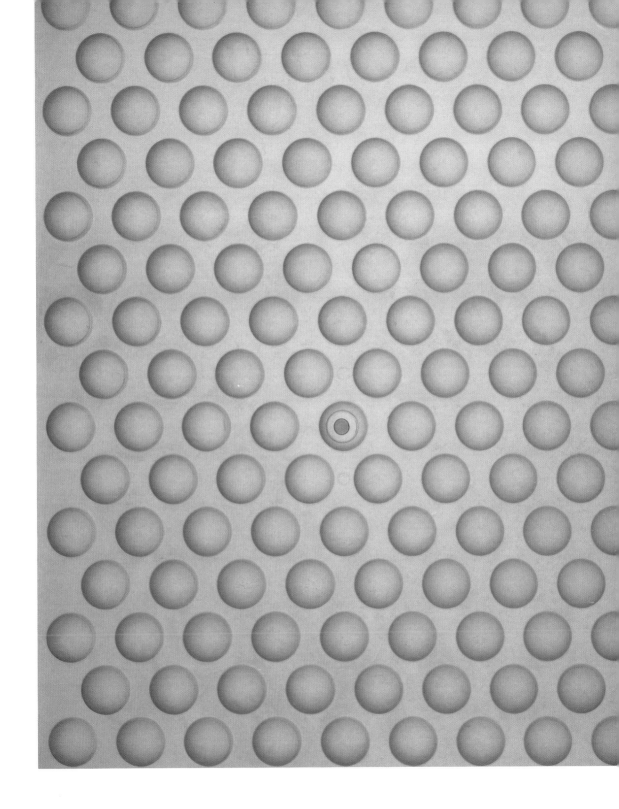

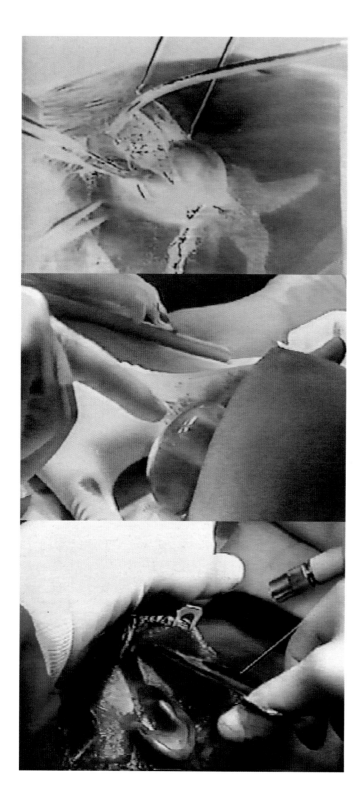

FOUR MINOR
RENOVATIONS:
REVAMP, REFURBISH,
RETOUCH, REFINE, 2000
Video
ARTIST Leora Farber, b. 1964

This video was produced by Leora Farber, an
artist whose work confronts contemporary
culture's obsession with reconstructing the
body. Here, Farber was permitted to
videotape a series of plastic surgeries. The
resulting video, which has a slow, soothing
musical score, is at once shockingly graphic
and strangely peaceful, revealing the
methodical care of the surgeon's art and the
malleability of the patient's body.

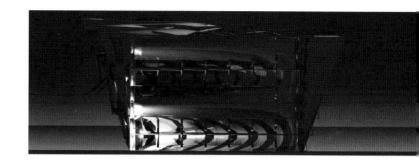

PARACUBE, 2001

Digital renderings

DESIGNER

Marcos Novak, b. 1957

Marcos Novak uses digital tools to create virtual architectural objects and spaces. His Paracube project shows a rectilinear structure whose flesh is pushing outward, engulfing and deforming the regular, Cartesian grid that would contain it. The interior membrane pulses outward, reshaping the outer frame.

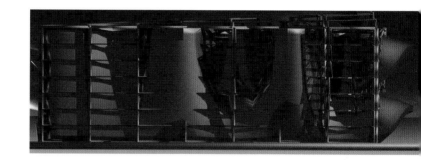

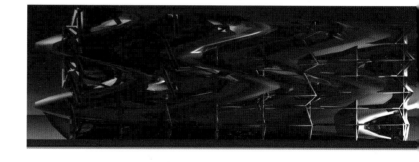

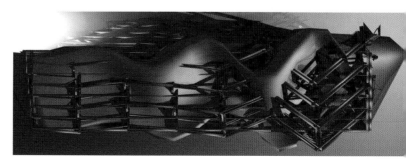

GEPETTO 2, GEPETTO 1, 1999
Photographs
PHOTOGRAPHY Margi Geerlinks, b. 1970
COURTESY OF Stux Gallery, New York

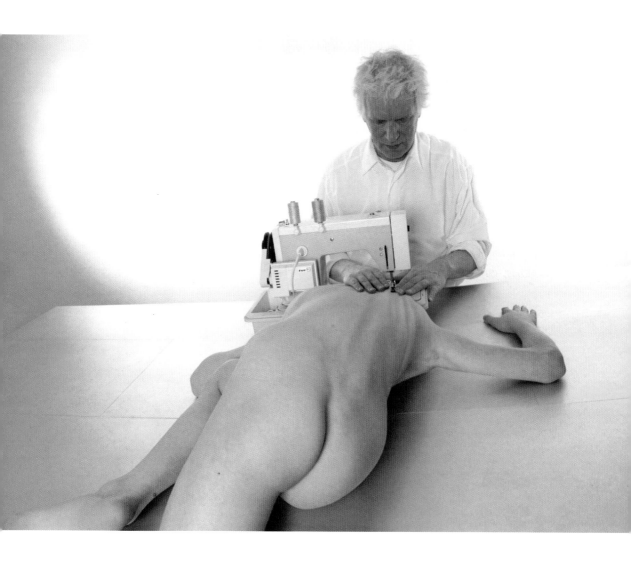

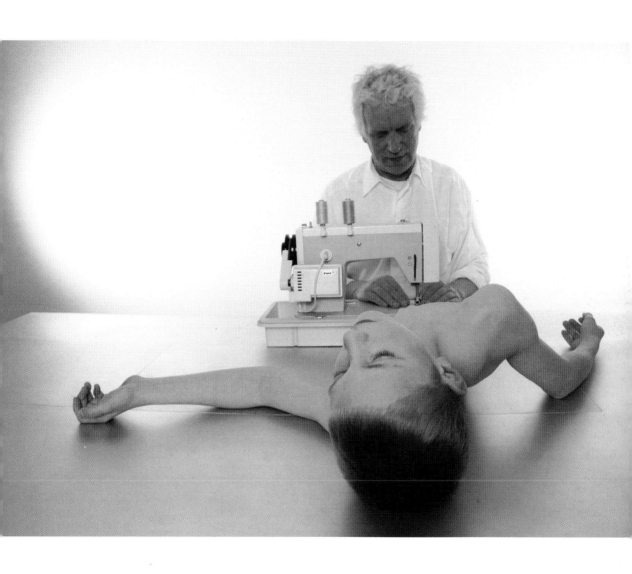

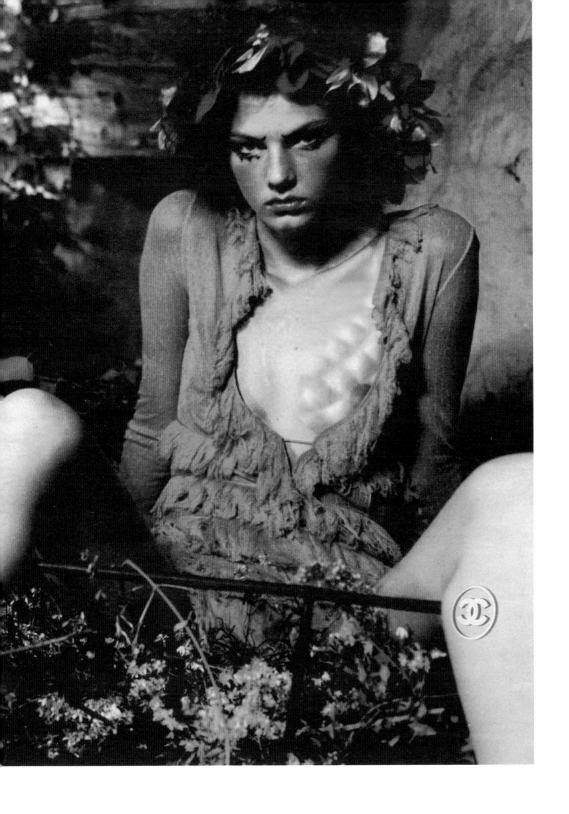

"As implant and explant technology become more sophisticated, and the idea of branding more intertwined into commodity culture, labels and bodies will become one. Whereas in the year 2000 we put labels on our bodies through the act of clothing, by 2020 we will be implanting designed body parts that not only are genetically coded but also bear the signs and brands of the couture and product houses that create them. Thus clothes will take on new function: not only will the protection aspect be far superior than what is available today, but physical exposures and protrusions will dictate the aesthetic of a line." —Carla Murray and Peter Allen

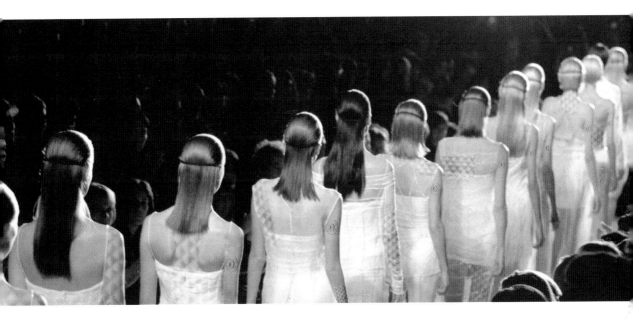

SKINTHETIC: CHANEL, 2001
Digital renderings
DESIGNERS Carla Murray, b. 1970
Peter Allen, b. 1968
KnoWear, Cataumet, Massachusetts

Skinthetic is a series of design proposals for "implant and explant" products that might in the future be used to extend consumer branding to the human body. Here, a quilted pattern derived from Chanel's brand identity is applied to the human torso. The skin of the garment becomes continuous with the skin of the body.

vessels
+
membranes

SKIN is a bag that holds in the organs and tissues of the body, a living luggage system. Contemporary bottles, bags, and garments combine natural and unnatural forms and materials, yielding objects that appear ripe with potential life.

Fashion clings to the body, becoming a surreal double, a nylon clone, or lives its own life, elaborating on natural anatomy with folds, growths, and protrusions. Buildings and bodies are clothed in surfaces that contradict the structures beneath. Materials such as glass and plastic become plump and pendulous.

An organ of the body, skin is a self-replacing surface with no clear boundaries. Some contemporary surfaces replicate the texture and porosity of natural skins, while others incorporate imagery and attributes alien to living things.

COVERED BELLY, 1997

Photograph

PHOTOGRAPHY   Elinor Carucci, b. 1971

COURTESY OF   Ricco/Maresca Gallery, New York

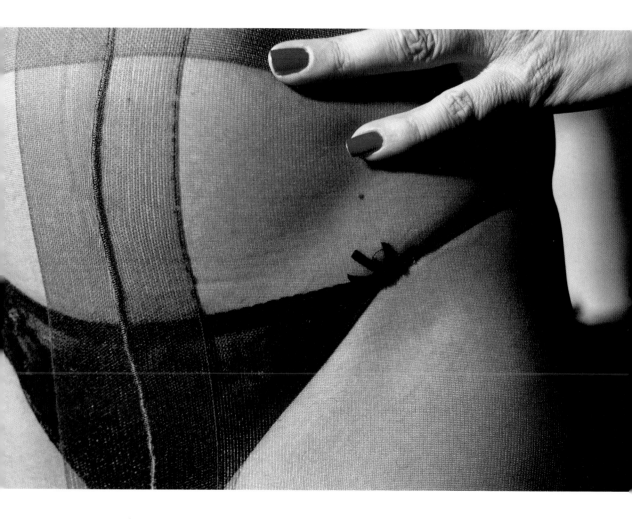

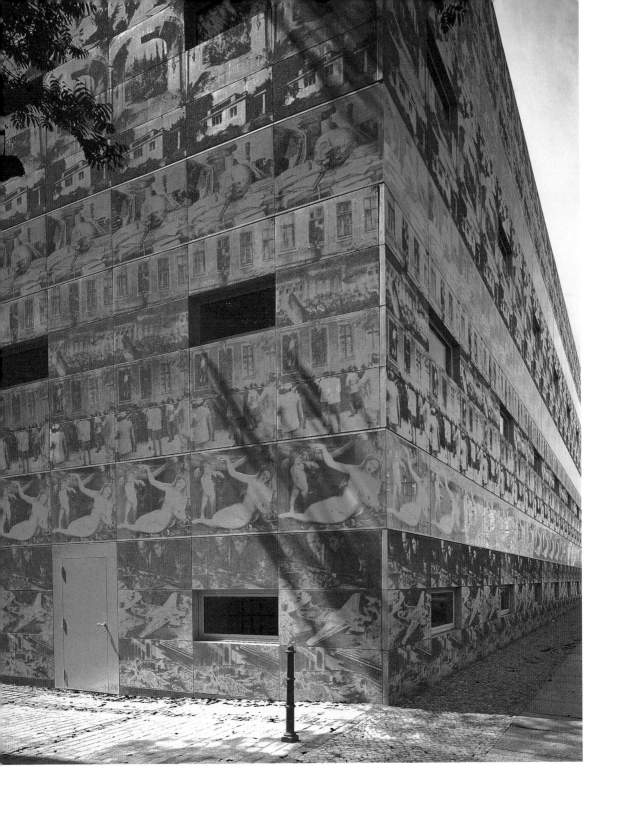

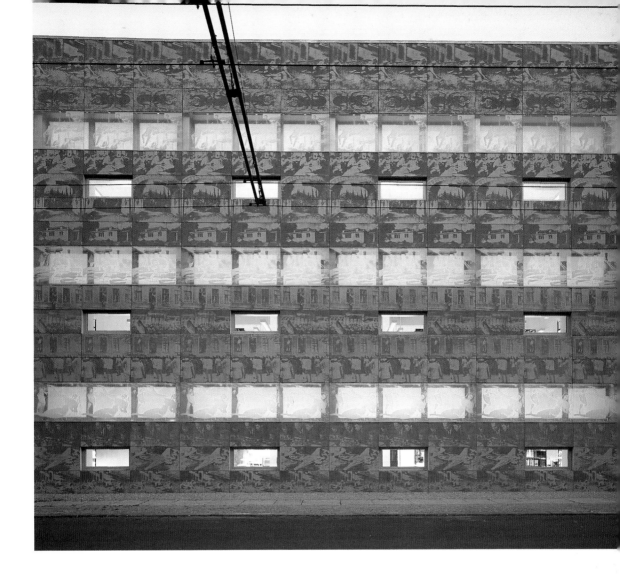

EBERSWALDE TECHNICAL SCHOOL
LIBRARY, EBERSWALDE, GERMANY, 1997–1999
ARCHITECTS Herzog & de Meuron, Switzerland
PARTNER IN CHARGE Pierre de Meuron, b. 1950
PROJECT ARCHITECTS Philippe Fürstenberger and Andreas Reuter
ENGINEERS GSE (structural); Dörner + Partners (climate control,
plumbing); Inginieure Büro Penke (electrical)
CONSULTANTS Betonsteinwerk Uetze (concrete); glazing (Fensterwelt)
PHOTOGRAPHY Margherita Spiluttini

Architects Jacques Herzog and Pierre de Meuron
focus on the condition of skins, layers, and shells
in their architecture. The exterior skins of their
buildings often are inscribed with imagery.
Their design for the Technical School Library in
Eberswalde, Germany, uses a serilith process to
transfer photographs to the building's concrete
surface. Images are also silkscreened directly onto
the glass. The result is a tattooed skin of glass
and concrete.

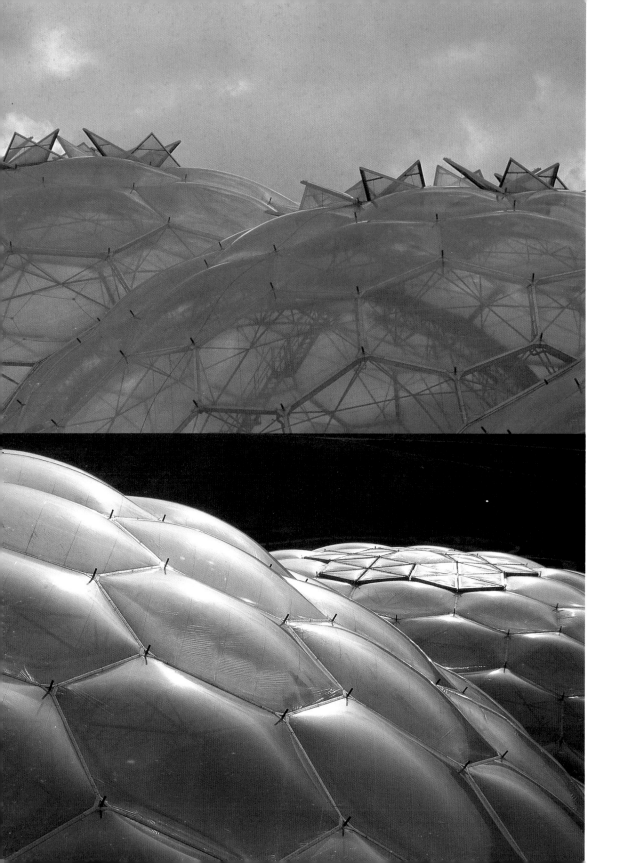

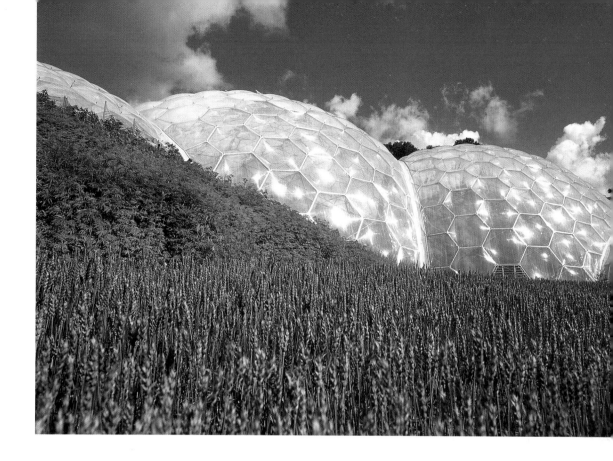

EDEN PROJECT

CORNWALL, UNITED KINGDOM, 2001

DESIGNERS Nicholas Grimshaw & Partners, United Kingdom

LANDSCAPE ARCHITECTS Land Use Consultants (Environmental Planning, Design, and Management)

STRUCTURAL ENGINEERS Anthony Hunt Associates

SERVICE ENGINEERS Ove Arup & Partners

QUANTITY SURVEYORS Davis Langdon & Everest

CONTRACTOR TEAM McAlpine Joint Venture

PHOTOGRAPHY Herbie Knott

The Eden Project, a millennium project dedicated to global biodiversity, is the largest plant enclosure in the world. Designed by Nicholas Grimshaw & Partners, the project's eight interlinked geodesic domes provide the maximum enclosed space within the minimum surface area. Each dome comprises two layers. The first is made of hexagonal steel modules that range in diameter from 5 to 11 meters. Each hexagon is assembled on the ground before it is craned into position and bolted to its neighbor by a standard cast-steel node. The first layer joins the second (inner) layer at these node points, the pinned connections guaranteeing structural stability. The domes are clad with ETFE (Ethylene Tetra Fluoro Ehtylene) foil, a lightweight material that is transparent to a wide spectrum of light. As such, it is suitable for a structure built to enclose developing plant life. It is also strong, antistatic, and recyclable, contributing to the overall realization of the Eden domes as tangible examples of energy-awareness in action.

"The space between the surface of the body and the surface of the skin—the interstitial territory bounding interior and exterior—allows each face of the building to alter as the light conditions change with the movements of the sun across the sky and of pedestrians along the street." —Thom Mayne, Morphosis

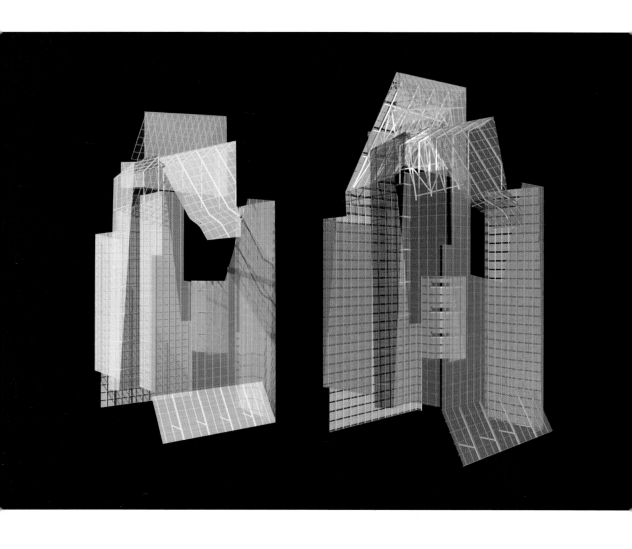

VILLAGE FASHION CENTER, SEOUL, KOREA, 1997

Digital renderings and photograph

DESIGNER Thom Mayne, b. 1944

Morphosis, Santa Monica, California

PHOTOGRAPHY Young-il Kim

In this building for a fashion school in Seoul, Morphosis designed
a building clad in a dramatic garment of translucent planes. A second
skin of perforated aluminum encloses the concrete volume of the
building. This fabriclike membrane is set 20 centimeters beyond the
interior body, creating a gap between inside and outside. The skin
is translucent by day and transparent by night, illuminated with light
from the interior.

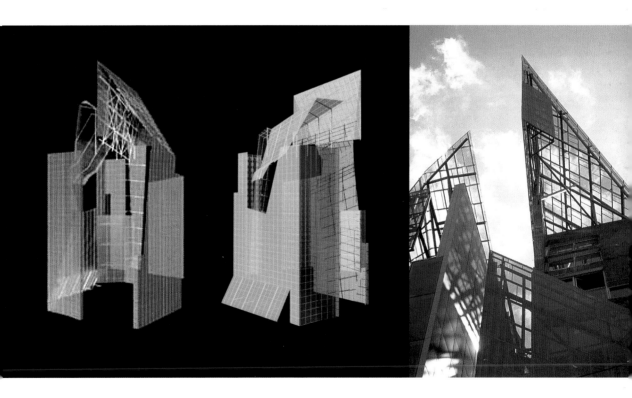

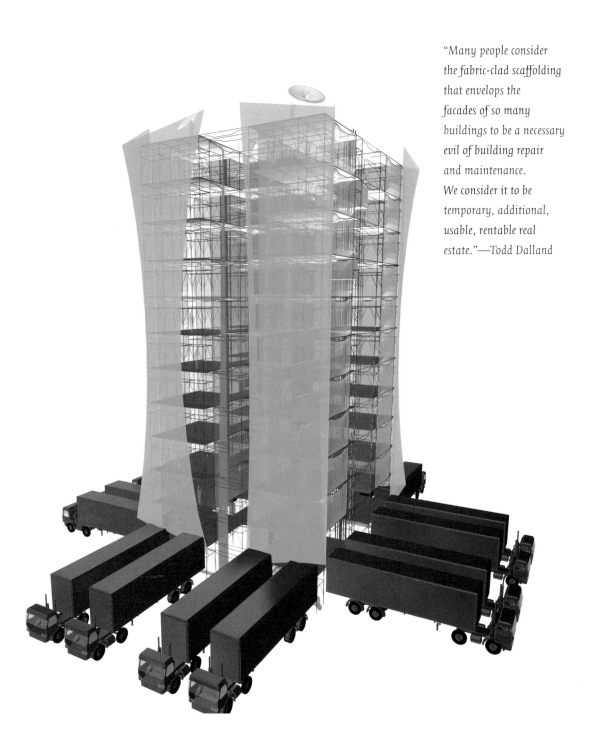

"Many people consider the fabric-clad scaffolding that envelops the facades of so many buildings to be a necessary evil of building repair and maintenance. We consider it to be temporary, additional, usable, rentable real estate."—Todd Dalland

RECYCLABLE, PORTABLE
SKYSCRAPER, 2001
Digital renderings

DESIGNERS Todd Dalland, b. 1951
Geza Gergo, b. 1973
Isamu Kanda, b. 1976
Tamer Onay, b. 1972
FTL Happold, New York

TEAM Megan Brothers, David Bott, Mary Korotkova,
Emily McDonald, Nestor Rave, Ashish Soni,
Numer Ybañez

FTL Happold is a firm specializing in the design and engineering of permanent and temporary tented and deployable structures. Proposed here is a portable, recyclable skyscraper, intended for temporary use on vacant urban sites for durations of six months to three years. This twelve-story building with forty-eight rental spaces has a total construction schedule of six weeks. The challenge was to create an entire building with scaffolding, standard clip-on floor planks, standard clip-on construction industry elevators, stackable event-industry toilets, and a double-layered fabric curtain wall. All of the infrastructure—power supply, water and waste lines, and mechanical systems—is housed in truck trailers occupying the first floor of the building at ground level. These components are standard, modular, and reusable—making the entire building recyclable. The building can be assembled on a flat site without foundations and still resist wind forces. Such a structure could help cities damaged by war or natural disaster.

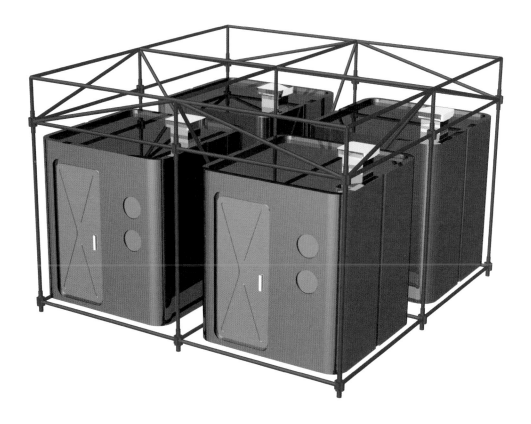

VILLA DALL'AVA, PARIS, 1991

Curtains, yellow and pink changeant silk

DESIGNER   Petra Blaisse, b. 1955

Inside Outside, Netherlands

PHOTOGRAPHY   © Frans Parthesius & Monica Hübner

Petra Blaisse has designed astonishing architectural curtains, as seen in her early project at the Villa dall'Ava, Paris. The proximity of neighboring villas made the wish for totally transparent facades problematic. In response, Blaisse designed a series of curtains and screens. In the living quarters downstairs, the silk curtains create a separate, enclosed space on the same level as the lawn outside. The glass walls in the corner of the space slide open in two directions, exposing the interior completely to the garden. The wind plays freely with the curtain, swinging the yellow silk from the inside out onto the lawn and back into the interior.

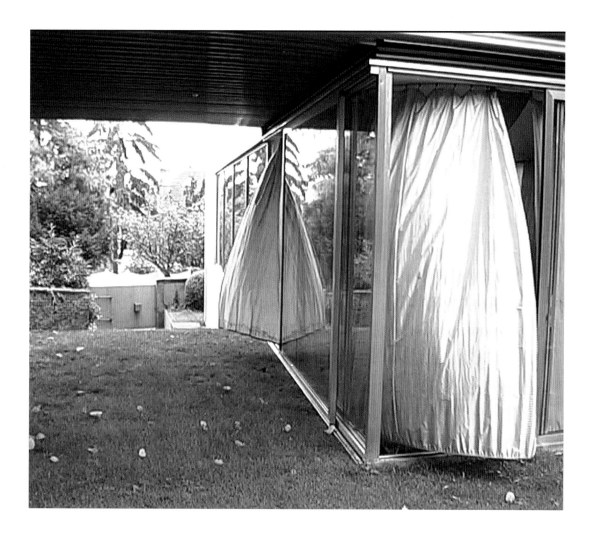

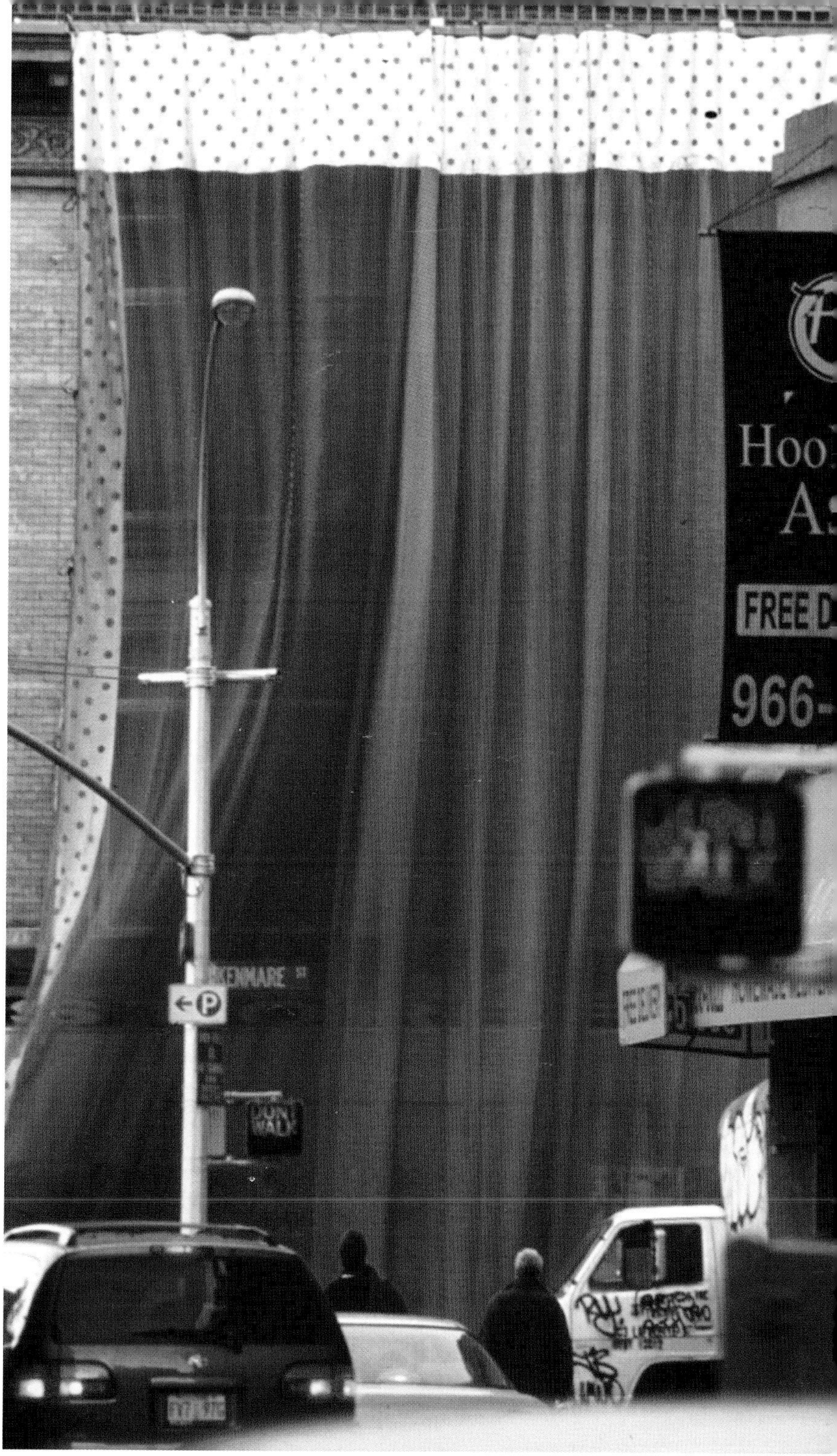

MOVEMENTS:
INTRODUCTION TO
A WORKING PROCESS,
NEW YORK, 2000
Curtain, yellow, red, and blue
scaffolding net, white
agricultural foil lined with
pink polyester
DESIGNER
Petra Blaisse
Inside Outside, Netherlands
Created for Storefront
for Art and Architecture,
New York
PHOTOGRAPHY
© Edgar Cleijne

Petra Blaisse created a
multistoried outdoor curtain
out of industrial fabrics for a
New York City exhibition
about her work. This
undulating, translucent
surface confronted the urban
setting with a jolt of lyricism.

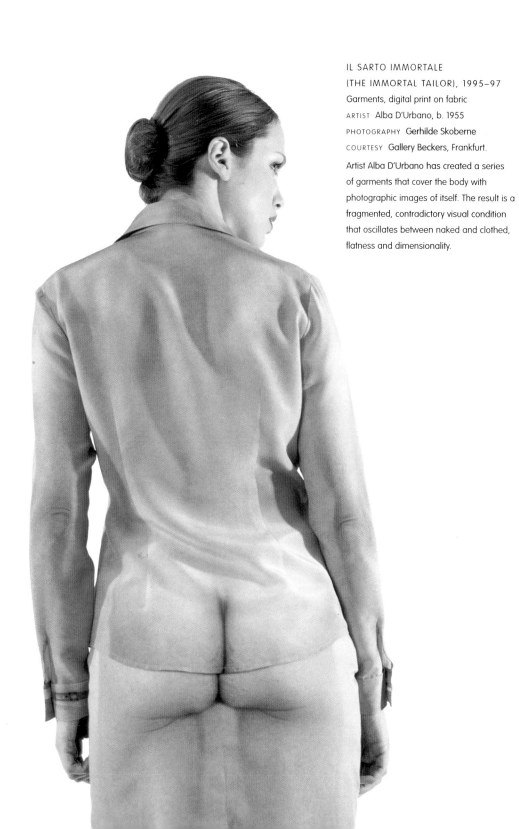

IL SARTO IMMORTALE
(THE IMMORTAL TAILOR), 1995–97
Garments, digital print on fabric
ARTIST Alba D'Urbano, b. 1955
PHOTOGRAPHY Gerhilde Skoberne
COURTESY Gallery Beckers, Frankfurt.

Artist Alba D'Urbano has created a series
of garments that cover the body with
photographic images of itself. The result is a
fragmented, contradictory visual condition
that oscillates between naked and clothed,
flatness and dimensionality.

"In order to realize the clothing of my own skin, I put photographs of my body into the computer digitally and then processed them, formed them, and cut them so that they fit into the dress-pattern of a suit. Thus it was possible to remodel the two-dimensional image into a three-dimensional body form in the tradition of the ancient art of tailors. The body becomes a virtual entity, a data landscape, a digital abstraction." —Alba D'Urbano

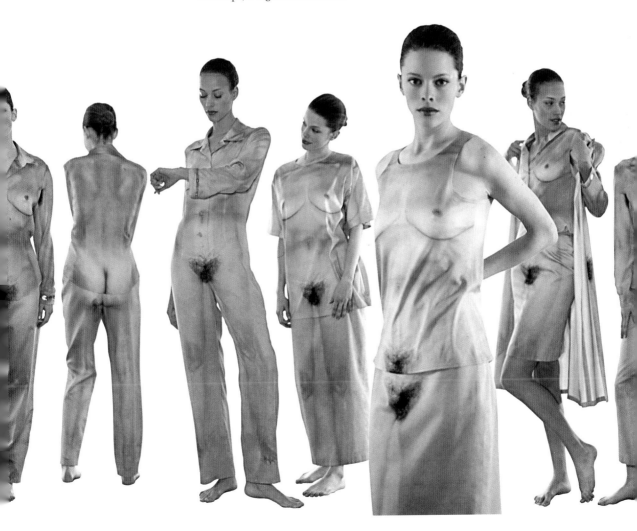

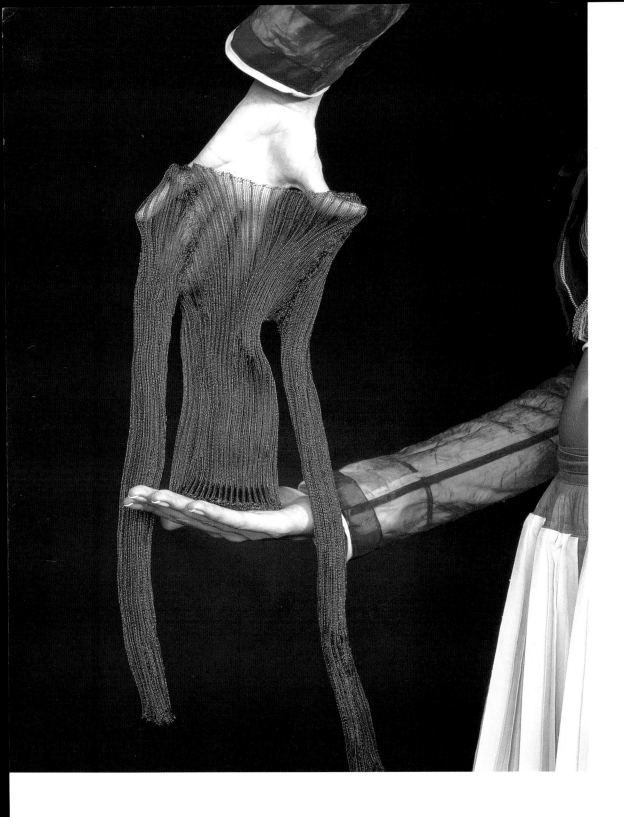

SERIE 100 BY STONE ISLAND
2001
Garments, nylon monofilament
DESIGNER Paul Harvey, b. 1957
Stone Island, Italy
MANUFACTURER
Sportswear Company S.P.A., Italy
PHOTOGRAPHY E/Marcus Gaab

This series of garments designed by
Paul Harvey for Stone Island are
constructed from an ultra-lightweight
nylon monofilament. Many of the
pieces are completely seamless.
Tiny when removed from the body,
they expand to fit the contours of the
wearer. The garments are designed to
be worn together; colors are muted
when viewed through layers. The
transparent gauze reveals the model as
well as the construction of the garment,
and can be worn over underwear
designed for display.

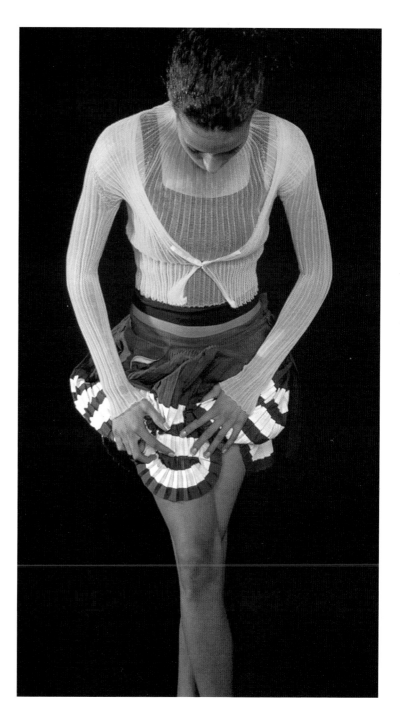

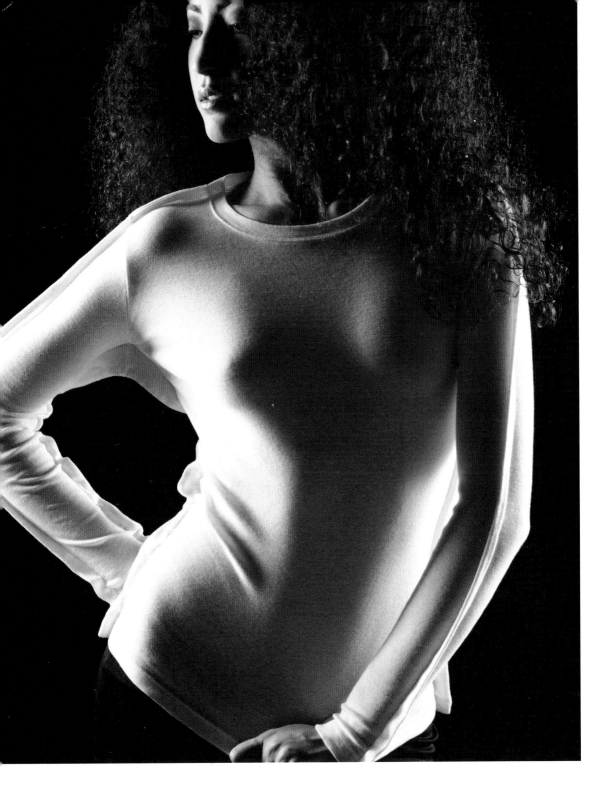

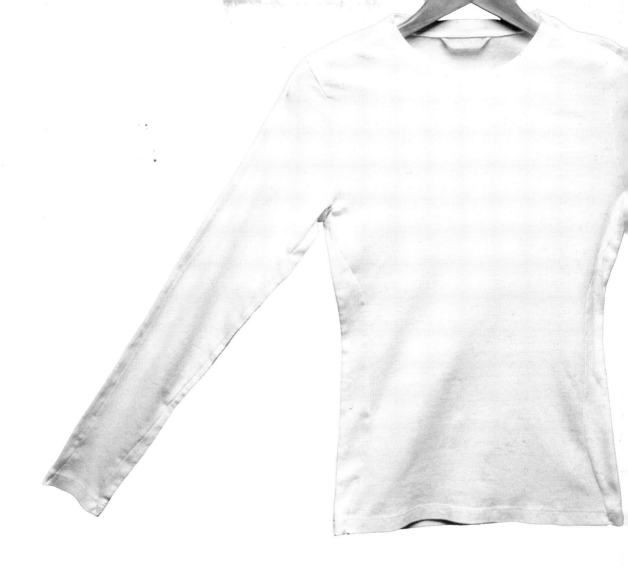

FITTED SHIRT, 2000

Cotton

DESIGNER Robert Stone, b. 1970

PHOTOGRAPHY Robert Stone

Los Angeles–based artist and architect
Robert Stone customizes t-shirts by
marking the shirt while it is on the wearer's
body, and then sewing the outline so
that the extra fabric remains outside the
new, close-fitting seam. A standard, mass-
produced shirt becomes a unique skin.·

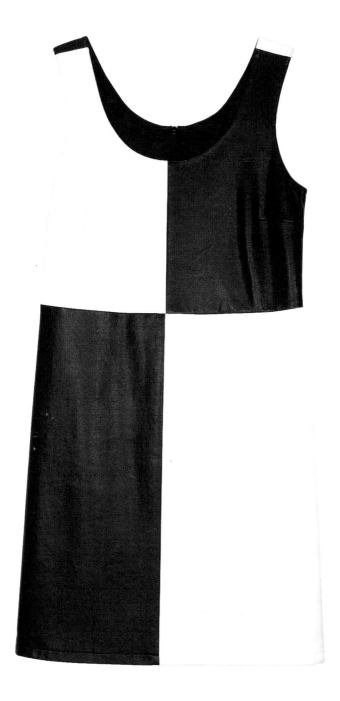

PLEATHER DRESS, 2000
Synthetic leather
DESIGNER Agnès B., Paris
PHOTOGRAPHY Dan Meyers

The French fashion house
Agnès B. here uses imitation
leather—an inexpensive
substitute known as
pleather—in a high-style
garment.

COW DRESS, 1999
Polyester fur and fleece, vinyl trim
DESIGNER The Gap, U.S.A.
PHOTOGRAPHY Dan Meyers

This child's dress incorporates a
variety of imitation animal skins,
from its fake cowhide exterior to
its vinyl trim and synthetic fleece
lining.

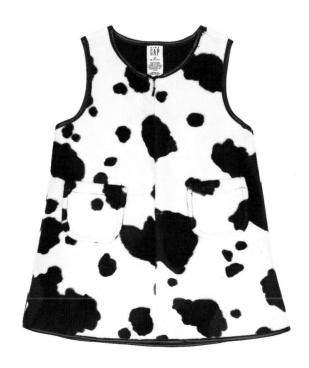

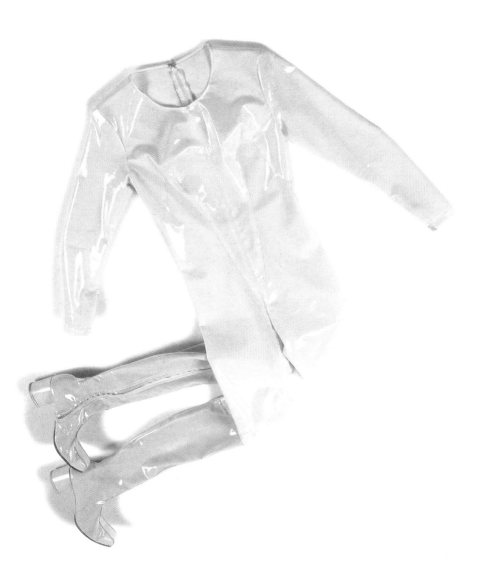

FUSE SECONDSKIN, 1997

Jumpsuit, light-sensitive PVC, zipper

INDUSTRIAL DESIGNER Yves Béhar, b. 1967

FASHION DESIGNER Angelita Tadeo, b. 1969

fuseproject, San Francisco

MANUFACTURER Jules and Jim, San Francisco

PHOTOGRAPHY Marcus Hanschen

Industrial designer Yves Béhar created this complete suit—including built-in shoes—out of shiny vinyl, recalling the flamboyant Pop fashions of the 1960s.

HUMAN FURRIER, 2000

Peach nipple handbags and shoes, silicone and leather

ARTIST Nicola Costantino, b. 1964

Manufactured in Argentina

COURTESY OF Deitch Projects, New York

The Argentine artist Nicola Costantino creates objects that comment on the meat and leather industries. In the surrealist tradition, these handbags and shoes are imprinted with tiny images of human nipples and anuses. Recalling the look of ostrich leather, the effect is at once decorative and alarming.

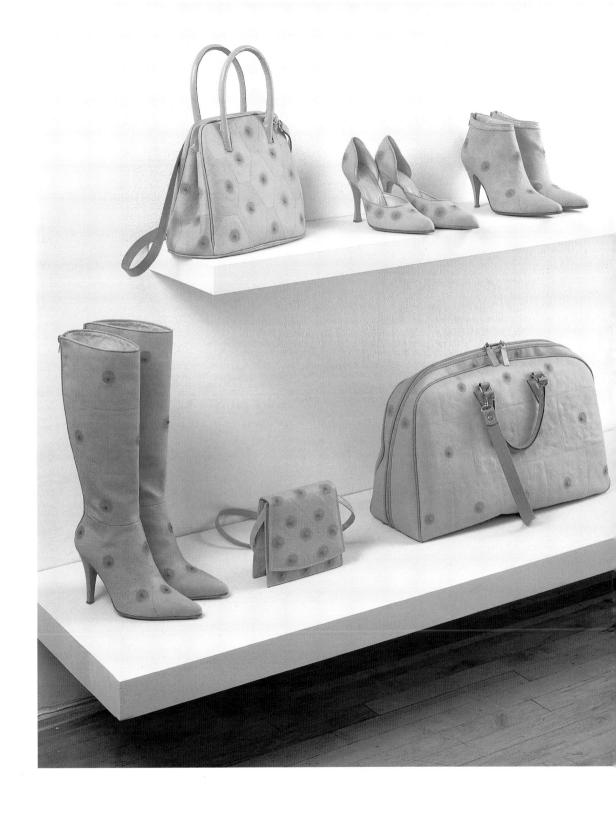

NIKE AIR HYPERFLIGHT (RIGHT)

Athletic shoe, synthetic upper, Phylon midsole,
exposed carbon fiber midfoot, rubber outsole
DESIGNER Eric Avar, b. 1968
MANUFACTURER Nike, Beaverton, Oregon

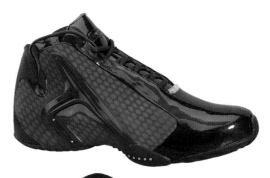

This Nike shoe aims to eliminate unnecessary
materials in order to create an ultra-lightweight
basketball shoe. Designer Eric Avar used the
least amount of rubber possible on the outsole,
kept the midsole low to the ground, and created
an unusual one-piece upper supported with
carbon fiber. The effect is a sleek, aerodynamic
skin for the foot.

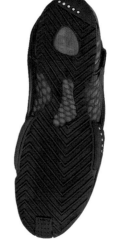

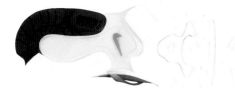

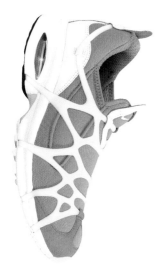

NIKE AIR KUKINI, 2000 (LEFT)

Athletic shoe, rubber outsole, Elastalon fit system (thermoplastic
urethane), OS meshler bootie (three-dimensionally woven
polyester), ethylene vinyl acetate midsole
DESIGNER Sean McDowell, b. 1971
MANUFACTURER Nike, Beaverton, Oregon

The upper of the Nike Air Kukini consists of a seamless stretch
mesh enclosed in an elastic "foot web" that keeps the shoe feeling
snug against the foot and replaces conventional laces.
The shoe becomes a second skin, married to the foot by a
translucent superstructure. The laceless design enables users to
quickly put on and remove the shoes, while visually the form
suggests an exotic organism emerging from an alien cocoon.

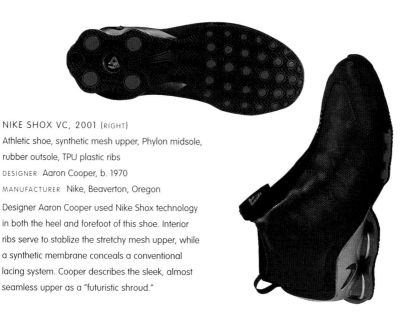

NIKE SHOX VC, 2001 (RIGHT)

Athletic shoe, synthetic mesh upper, Phylon midsole, rubber outsole, TPU plastic ribs

DESIGNER Aaron Cooper, b. 1970

MANUFACTURER Nike, Beaverton, Oregon

Designer Aaron Cooper used Nike Shox technology in both the heel and forefoot of this shoe. Interior ribs serve to stablize the stretchy mesh upper, while a synthetic membrane conceals a conventional lacing system. Cooper describes the sleek, almost seamless upper as a "futuristic shroud."

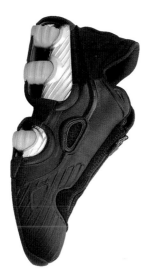

NIKE SHOX XT, 2001 (LEFT)

Athletic shoe, synthetic leather uppers, polyurethane columns, TPU plastic midsole, solid rubber outsole

DESIGNERS Nike Crosstraining design team

MANUFACTURER Nike, Beaverton, Oregon

This Nike Shox system returns energy to its user's jump. The design exposes the shoe's interior anatomy, drawing attention to the Shox mechanism.

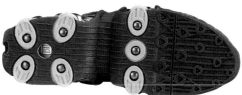

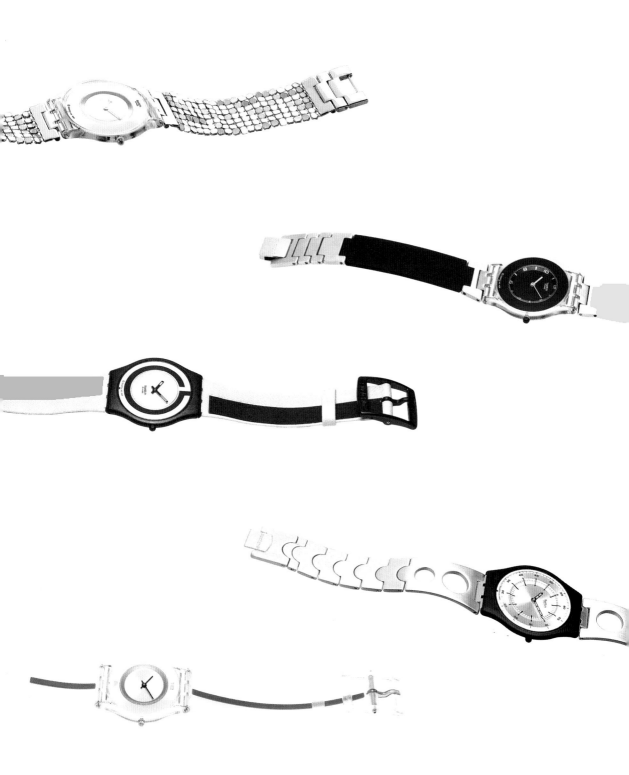

SWATCH SKIN COLLECTION

Watches, various materials

DESIGNERS Swatch Design Team

MANUFACTURER Swatch Group of Switzerland

Swatch's Skin Collection features an extremely thin watch mechanism housed in a variety of faces with coordinating bands in diverse materials. Some of the watches feature translucent plastic that reveals the internal mechanism as well as the skin of the wearer. Others use metal, rubber, or vinyl in designs that recall traditional jewelry styles in a stylized, technology-inflected manner. By using minimal materials in an openly expressive way, Swatch's Skin Collection treats the watch both as functional jewelry and as expressive fashion accessory.

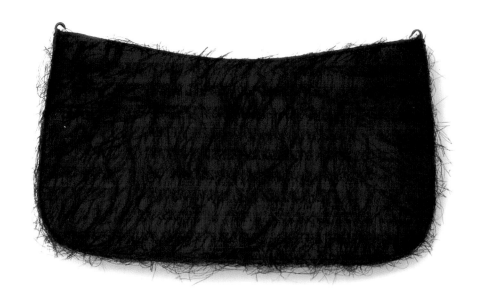

THREAD BAG, 2000
Handbag, nylon, leather
DESIGNER Kenneth Cole, b. 1954
MANUFACTURER Kenneth Cole Reaction
PHOTOGRAPHY Dan Meyers

Threads of nylon emerge across the surface of this microfiber handbag. Longer than human body hairs and more sparse than animal fur, the strands of thread invoke the skin of an anomalous being.

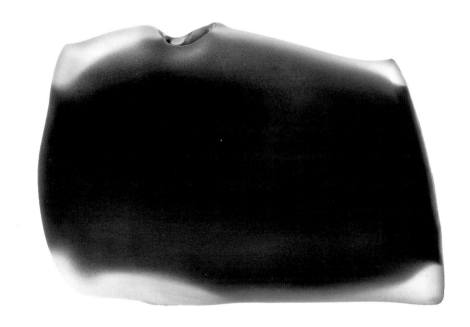

STONE, 2001

Glass vase

DESIGNER   Adam Aaronson, 1956

MANUFACTURER   Aaronson Noon, United Kingdom

PHOTOGRAPHY   Dan Meyers

English glassmaker Adam Aaronson has made a densely opaque object out of a material typically prized for its transparency and lightness. The opening in the vase is made after the piece is blown, whereas in the conventional method, the opening originates where air enters the molten material. In Aaronson's piece, the enclosed pocket of glass is made by closing together the ends; the opening is then cut into the side—an incision in glass flesh.

TWIN, 2000
Vessel, Murano glass
DESIGNER Nigel Coates, b. 1949
Part of *Salviati Meets London*, exhibition
curated by Vessel Gallery, London
Collection of Adrian Price, United Kingdom
MANUFACTURER Salviati, Italy
PHOTOGRAPHY Vessel Gallery, London

Whereas traditonal glass vases are upright and symmetrical,
these droop and hang in an embodied way, bumping
against each other like a pair of breasts or testicles.
The vases are pendulous rather than perky, and have a
liquid, elastic appearance.

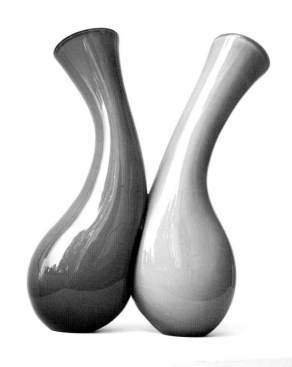

PHILOU, 2000

Vessel, blow-molded LDPE, ABS, ink

DESIGNER Yves Béhar, b. 1967

fuseproject, San Francisco

GRAPHIC DESIGN Yves Béhar, Palm Kulapongse

MANUFACTURER Philou Inc., U.S.A.

PHOTOGRAPHY Marcus Hanschen

To package these hair-care products for the teen market, Yves Béhar created a form based on a tilted oval. A gentle angle animates the bottle, making it appear changeable, caught in a slow-motion transformation. One side is narrower for smaller hands to grip, and the object feels soft but solid to the touch, like young skin.

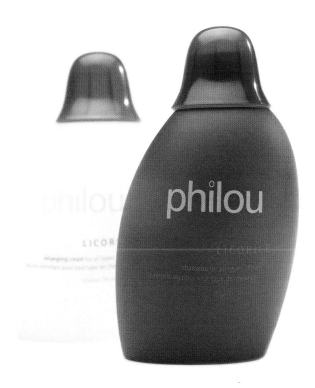

EGG VASE, 1997

Vase, porcelain

DESIGNER Marcel Wanders, b. 1963

Marcel Wanders Studio, Netherlands

MANUFACTURER Moooi, Netherlands

Droog Design Collection

PHOTOGRAPHY Maarten van Houten

The molds for Marcel Wanders's Egg vases are made by stuffing a condom with eggs. Cast in bright white porcelain, the resulting objects are at once organic and hygienic, as the fertile form of the eggs presses against the protective sheath.

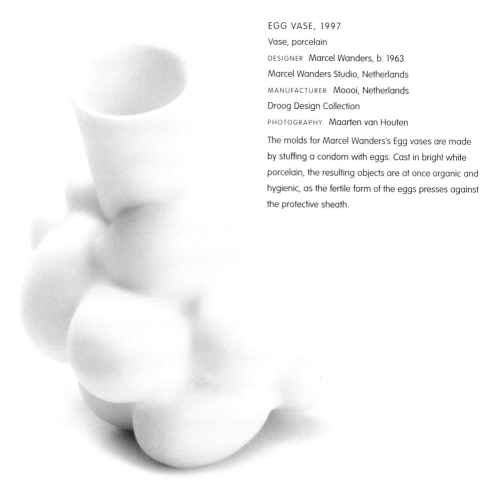

AIRBORNE SNOTTY VASE:

SINUSITUS, 2001

Vase, polyamide

DESIGNER Marcel Wanders

Marcel Wanders Studio, Netherlands

MANUFACTURER Cappellini, Italy

PHOTOGRAPHY Maarten van Houten

Wanders's Airborne Snotty Vase series is based on a 3d-scan of the microscopic components of a human airborne sneeze. Using a microtech imaging device, the sneezes—produced by people suffering from the diseases influenza, ozaena, pollinosis, sinusitus, and coryza—are transformed into solid representations.

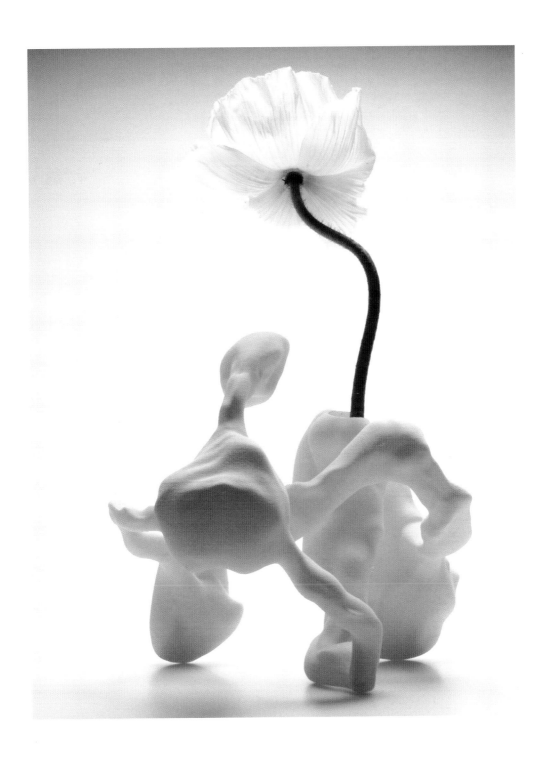

FOAM BOWL, 1997
Porcelain bowl
DESIGNER Marcel Wanders, b. 1963
Marcel Wanders Studio, Netherlands
Studio Marcel Wanders
Droog Design
MANUFACTURER Moooi, Netherlands
PHOTOGRAPHY Maarten van Houten

This bowl by Marcel Wanders is made by dipping a sponge into liquid porcelain. When the dipped sponge is fired in a kiln, the sponge burns away, leaving only the porcelain. The result is a hard, rigid object with an open, porous skin.

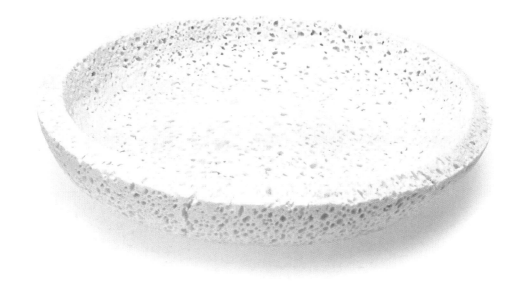

QUEEN ANNE'S LACE, 2000

Tea strainer, silver

DESIGNER   Ted Muehling, b. 1953

MANUFACTURER   Ted Muehling, New York

PHOTOGRAPHY   Dan Howell

This tea strainer by Ted Muehling is made by etching holes into a thin sheet of silver. Minimal material is used to create an almost liquid, bubbling surface.

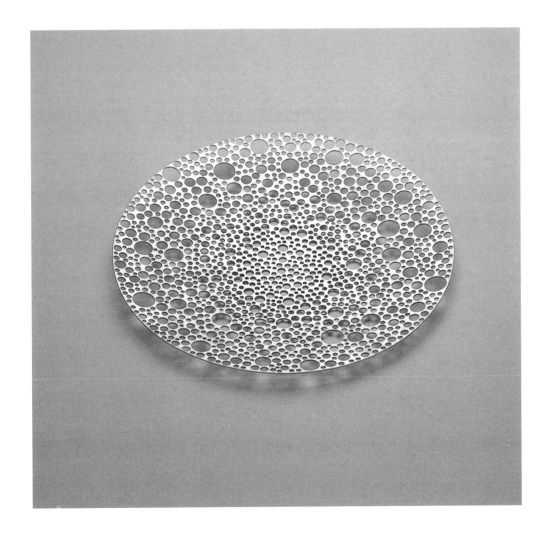

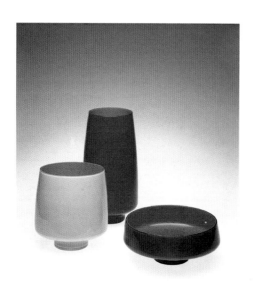

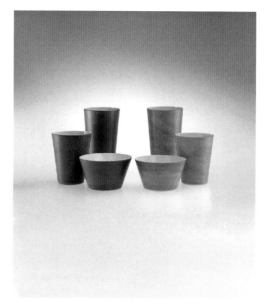

CARIOCA, 1998 (LEFT)
MARMORATI, 2000 (RIGHT)
Vases, glass
DESIGNER Rodolfo Dordoni, b. 1954 (Carioca)
MANUFACTURER Venini, Italy

These vases, produced by the famous Venetian glassmaker
Venini, feature double layers of glass, one blown over the
other—two skins of contrasting colors.

DESKTOP LANDSCAPES: INFINITY, SOUL,
CUBE, AND RIBBON, 1999
Vases, vinyl dipped PVC
DESIGNER Karim Rashid, b. 1960
MANUFACTURER Totem, New York

These flexible containers by Karim Rashid are
made by dipping the mold twice into a liquid
material, once for each color. The result of this
simple process is soft vessels that shift color
from top to bottom or inside to outside.

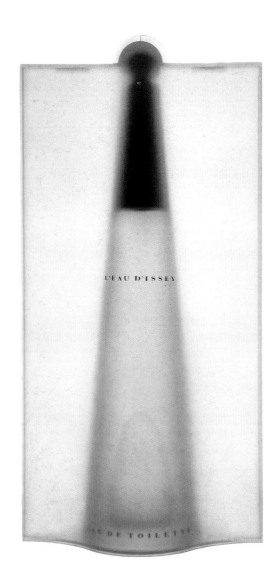

L'EAU D'ISSEY, 1999
Package, glass, metal
DESIGNER Karim Rashid, b. 1960
MANUFACTURER Issey Miyake, Japan
PHOTOGRAPHY Ilan Rubin

Karim Rashid's fragrance bottle for
Issey Miyake consists of flat planes of
frosted glass that swell around the
vessel of liquid within.

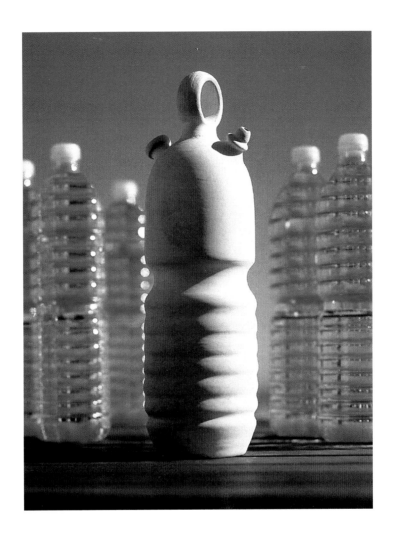

SIESTA, 2000
Bottle, white terra cotta
DESIGNERS Alberto Martinez, b. 1974
Raky Martinez, b. 1973
Héctor Serrano, b. 1974
MANUFACTURER La Mediterranea, Spain

Siesta, a terra cotta vessel for water, combines the look of mass-produced plastic bottles with the functional advantages of a traditional *botijo*, used for carrying drinking water in Spain. The special white terra cotta keeps water cold, even in direct sun. The Siesta is made by hand in Spain, using the same techniques as the *botijo*.

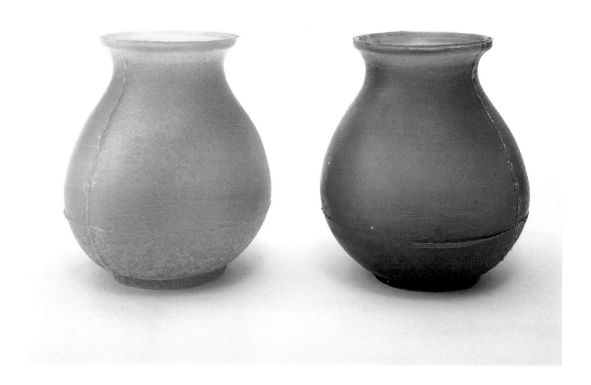

PINK AND NATURAL SOFT URN
1999, 1994
Vases, soft polyurethane
DESIGNER   Hella Jongerius, b. 1963
MANUFACTURER Hella Jongerius, Netherlands
PHOTOGRAPHY   Bob Goedewaagen

These soft vases by Hella Jongerius assume a classical shape but are rendered in an untraditional material. With Natural Urn (right), Jongerius sought to make plastic—a material associated with youth and newness—feel old, showing scratches, bubbles, and seams from the molding process. Pink Urn (left) was made later from the same mold, but from fresh, pink silicone.

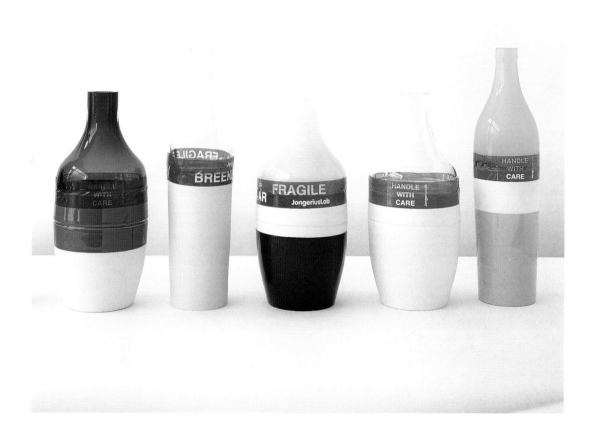

GROOVE AND LONG NECK
2000
Bottles, porcelain, glass, tape
DESIGNER   Hella Jongerius
MANUFACTURER   Hella Jongerius, Netherlands
PHOTOGRAPHY   Bob Goedewaagen

This series of bottles by Jongerius combines found elements and new materials. The continuous skin of traditional containers gives way to an assembly of diverse parts: glass bottles are joined with tape to ceramic bases.

"Instead of having the pure perfume slushing around in a clear bottle, we confined it to a precious area while surrounding it with an oversized clear mass."
—Yves Béhar

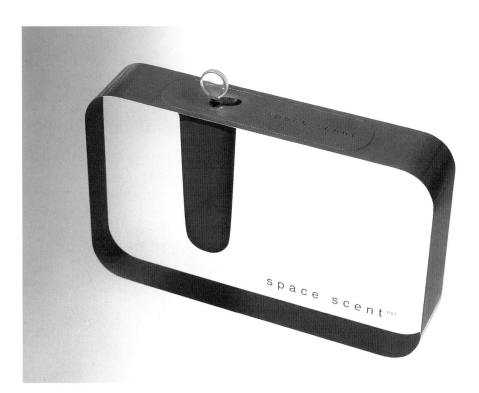

space scent

SPACE SCENT, 2000
Vessel, polyurethane resin, polyurethane elastomer, ink

DESIGNERS Yves Béhar, b. 1967
Johan Liden, b. 1974
fuseproject, San Francisco

CASTING ADVISOR Corey Jones

MANUFACTURER Spaceprojekt, Brent Haas, San Francisco

PHOTOGRAPHY Alan Purcell

With his design for the Space Scent bottle, Yves Béhar has shifted the conventional relationship between container and space. The larger, clear bottle area is solid, while the perfume cavity is opaque and visually connected to the red edge outlining the object.

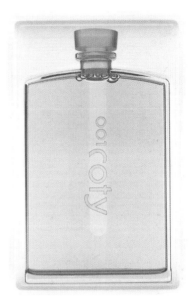

001COTY, 2001
Fragrance bottle and packaging
Glass, thermoplastic elastomer

DESIGN CONCEPT Coty Inc.
PACKAGE DESIGN Dan Lewis, Lewis Design+Planning
Brennan Liston
FRAGRANCE Jim Krivda, Fragrance Resources, New York
LOGO DESIGN David Shields
MANUFACTURERS Pochet, France (bottle)
Lombardi Design and Manufacturing,
New York (case)
PHOTOGRAPHY Shoot Digital

To create this limited-edition fragrance and packaging, Coty sought to reflect the convergence of bodies and technology. The flask, modeled on a simple, modern design from 1917, is enclosed within a flexible skin made from the same type of plastic used to cover prosthetic limbs. The unisex fragrance is intended to evoke the smell of electricity, the scent of digital information.

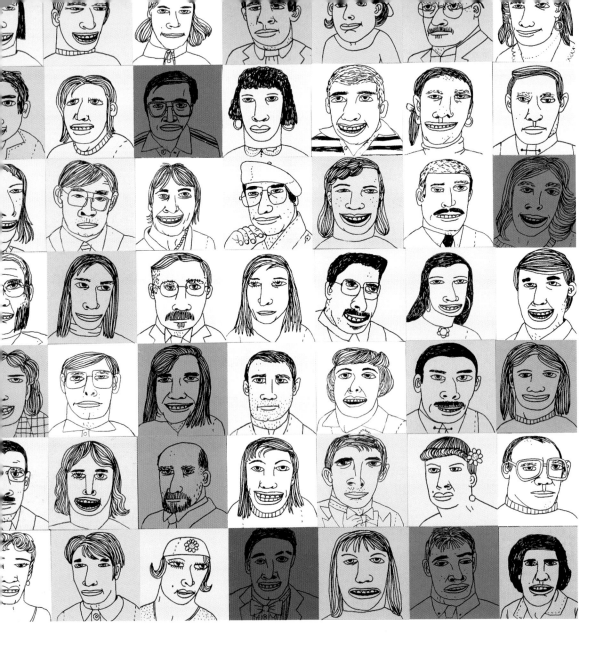

MILLENNIUM COLLECTION: YEARBOOK, 1999
Design for decorative high-pressure laminate (HPL)
DESIGNER Mark Todd, b. 1970
Millennium Collection curated by
Grace Jeffers
MANUFACTURER Wilsonart International, U.S.A.

The laminate surface company Wilsonart
issued its Millennium Collection in 1999, a
series of experimental patterns created by
artists and designers.

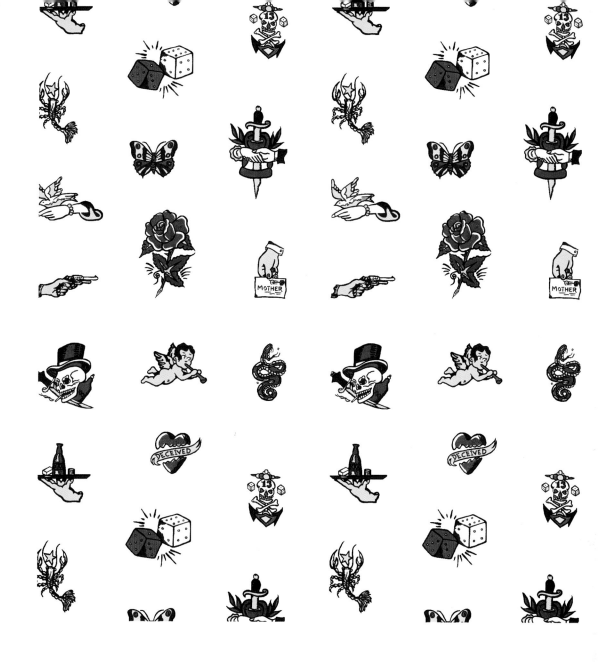

MILLENNIUM COLLECTION: FLASH, 1999
Design for decorative high-pressure laminate (HPL)
DESIGNER   Christine Scholtz, b. 1963
Millennium Collection curated by
Grace Jeffers
MANUFACTURER   Wilsonart International, U.S.A.

This surface from Wilsonart's Millennium
Collection incorporates designs used by
tattoo artists.

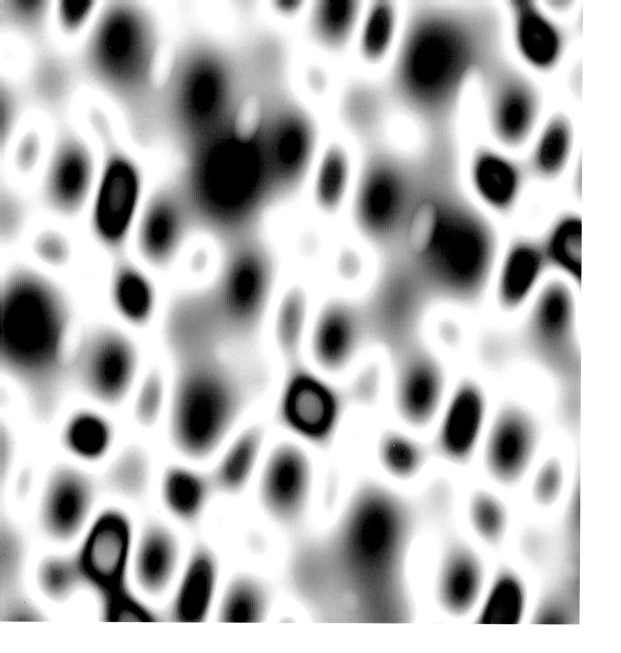

MILLENNIUM COLLECTION: SLOW, 1999
Design for decorative high-pressure laminate (HPL)
DESIGNER Michael Solis, b. 1969
Millennium Collection curated by
Grace Jeffers
MANUFACTURER Wilsonart International, U.S.A.

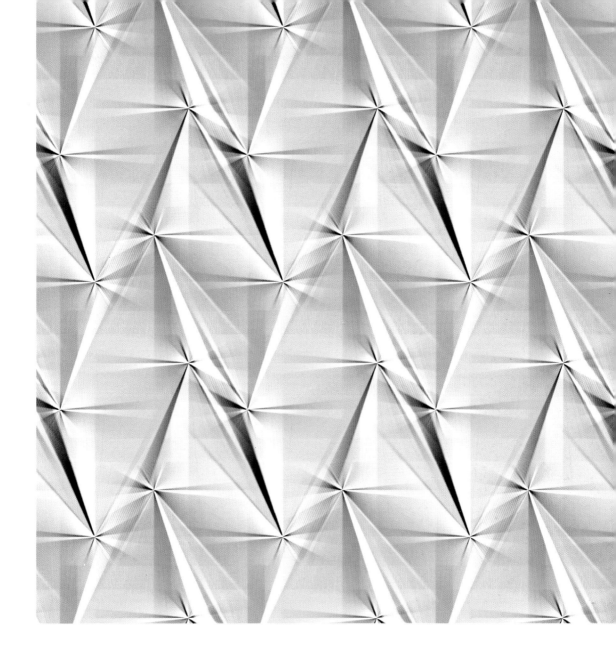

CREASE, 2000
Pattern

DESIGNERS Rhona Nam-Pijja, b. 1973
James Bullen, b. 1968
Bullen.Pijja Design Ltd., London

MANUFACTURER Stock Printers, Netherlands

PHOTOGRAPHY John Juniper

Bullen.Pijja's Crease, a pattern designed to be printed on fabric, creates the illusion of wrinkles within an overtly regular repeat. Printed digitally, the pattern is reproduced in fine detail, heightening the illusion.

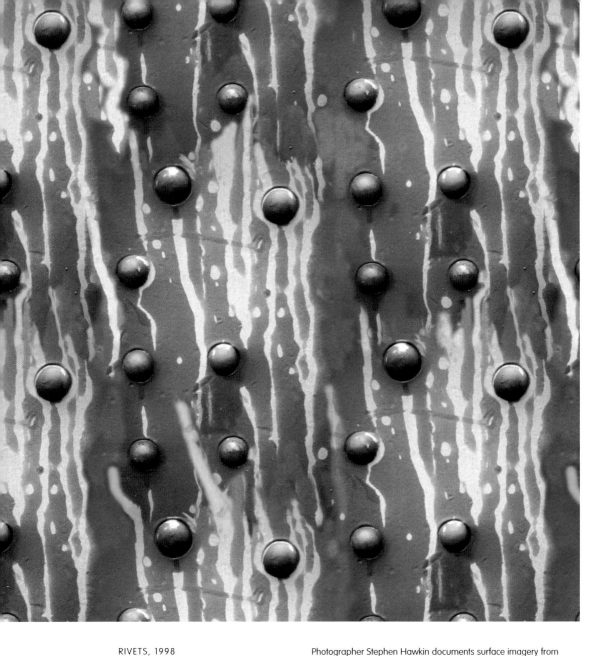

RIVETS, 1998

Photograph, laminate

DESIGNER   Stephen Hawkin, b. 1965

Stephen Hawkin Design

MANUFACTURER   Wilsonart, U.S.A.

Photographer Stephen Hawkin documents surface imagery from Scotland's industrial and nautical landscape. Some of his photographs have been made into custom laminates. This pattern was produced as a custom laminate by Wilsonart specially for the Skin project. Working with a photograph of a bridge at Leith Docks, Edinburgh, Hawkin digitally constructed a pattern that repeats across a large area. The resulting image—at once regular and irregular, organic and technological—celebrates the impact of time and weather on an industrial skin.

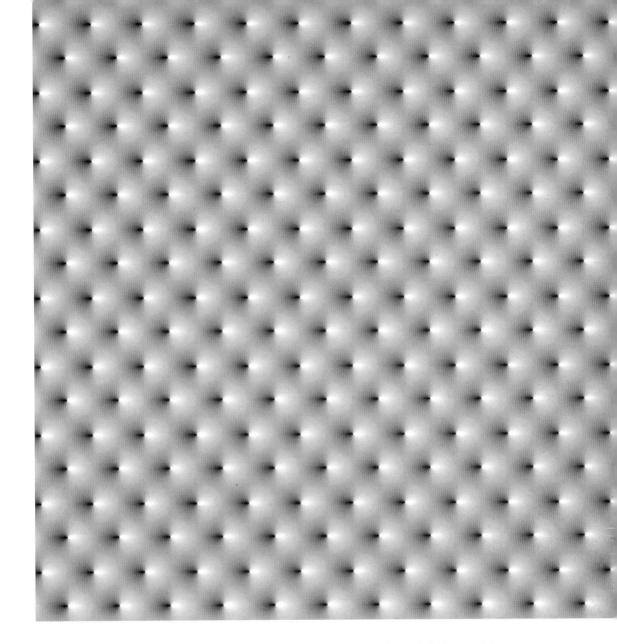

BUMPS, 2000
Design for digitally printed fabric

DESIGNERS Rhona Nam-Pijja, b. 1973
James Bullen, b. 1968
Bullen.Pijja Design Ltd., London

MANUFACTURER Stock Printers, Netherlands

PHOTOGRAPHY John Juniper

Rhona Nam-Pijja and James Bullen have created a series of patterns that combine naturalistic forms— wrinkles, bulges, dimples—into patently artificial, overtly modular designs. The patterns are printed on laminates and fabrics, enabling planar surfaces to appear at once 2d and 3d. Bullen.Pijja's surfaces harbor an illusion of depth that is ominous and uncanny, rendered with photographic precision via digital design and printing techniques.

intelligence
+
touch

SKIN is the body's largest sense organ, registering warmth and cold, pleasure and pain, and an infinite array of textures. The skins of objects, buildings, and garments today respond to input from users and the environment, from shifts in temperature or light to digitally acquired information.

Skin is the plane of contact between people and things. The skins of mechanical and electronic devices are the point of interface with users; their surfaces convey the identity of an object and contain its controls. In the 1920s and 1930s, the pioneers of industrial design created hard shells around the mechanical "guts" of appliances. Today, designers construct skins for objects that are warmer, more responsive to the touch. Devices are increasingly controlled by screen-based interfaces as well as physical buttons and keypads. Thousands of interface "skins" can be downloaded from the Web, allowing users to create and exchange digital controls.

HAND IN BATHROOM, 1996
Photograph
PHOTOGRAPHY Elinor Carucci, b. 1971
COURTESY OF Ricco/Maresca Gallery, New York

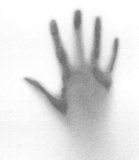

DIVISUMMA 18, 1972

Electronic printing calculator

ABS plastic, melamine, rubber

DESIGNER Mario Bellini, b. 1935

COLLECTION OF Cooper-Hewitt, National Design
Museum, Smithsonian Institution, 1986.99.41

MANUFACTURER Olivetti, Italy

PHOTOGRAPHY Matt Flynn

When Mario Bellini designed this calculator for Olivetti in 1972, he fundamentally expanded the paradigm of industrial design. In place of the hard, often glossy shells that designers had constructed around mechanical objects since the 1920s, Bellini created a soft rubber skin. The mechanical keys press up through the taut, elastic surface.

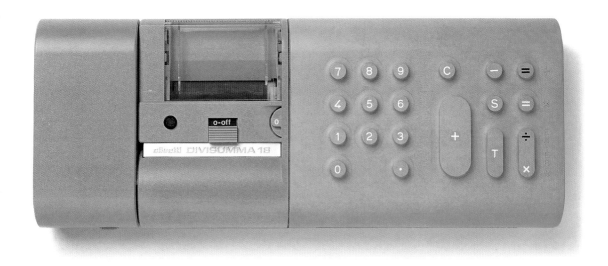

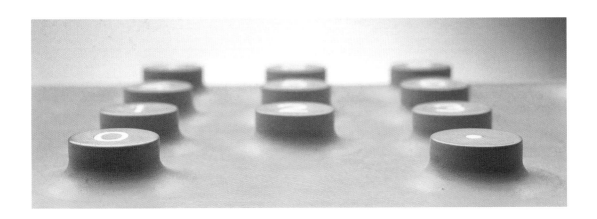

ELEKTEX SOFT KEYBOARD, 2001

Keyboard, pressure formed ElekTex (conductive textile) on siliconized foam, rubberized silicone with IR transmission capability, electronic components

DESIGNER   Sam Hecht, b. 1969
                IDEO, United Kingdom
MANUFACTURER   ElectroTextiles, United Kingdom
PHOTOGRAPHY   Richard Davis

The industrial design firm IDEO has worked with ElectroTextiles to develop uses for ElekTex, a conductive fabric that can sense the location and pressure of human touch. Whereas Bellini stretched a neutral membrane around mechanical parts, the ElekTex skin is an active surface, a sensing and switching system that translates electronic impulses into digital data. When a user touches it, ElekTex recognizes the contact point and sends signals to various devices, such as a CPU or a VCR. The fabric is made from a combination of conductive fibers and common textile fibers. It is flexible, waterproof, programmable, and inexpensive to produce.

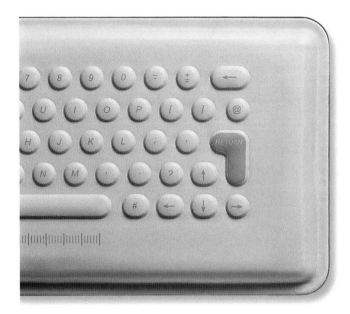
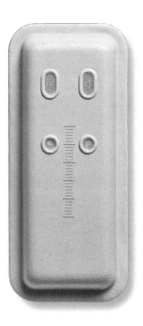

BOB-BOT, 2001

Computer game, prototype

DESIGNERS Eric Arcacha, b. 1978

J. Philip Newsanger, b. 1973

The field of game design is populated with countless cyborgs, intelligent beings who incorporate technological and organic components. This prototype for a children's game invites the user to assemble a bionic baby out of a kit of alien parts. The baby then battles an equally imposing enemy, constructed by the game.

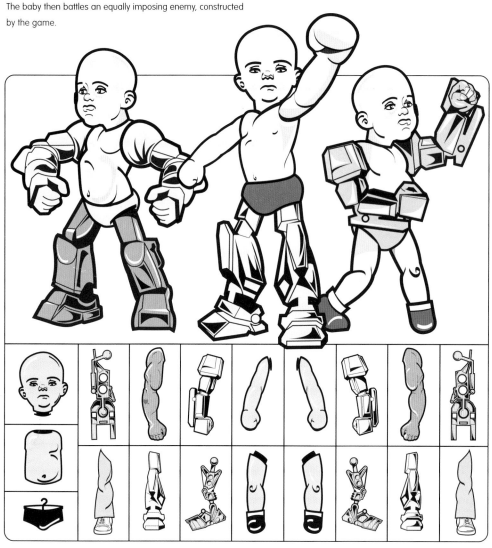

SIMS SKIN, 2001

DESIGNER Elke Gasselseder, b. 1976

The Sims is a computer game in which a player assembles a digital family and their household; the player then participates as the characters evolve and interact, sometimes disastrously. Social relationships are simulated in response to various factors, such as the compatibility of the characters and their economic circumstances. An amateur subculture is devoted to creating custom "skins," or characters, for The Sims game. A designer creates a flat image using software such as PhotoShop; the resulting surface is then wrapped around a 3d model for use within the game environment. The skin shown here wears a pleather dress by Agnès B. and Nike Air Kikuni shoes.

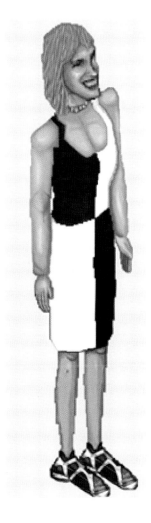

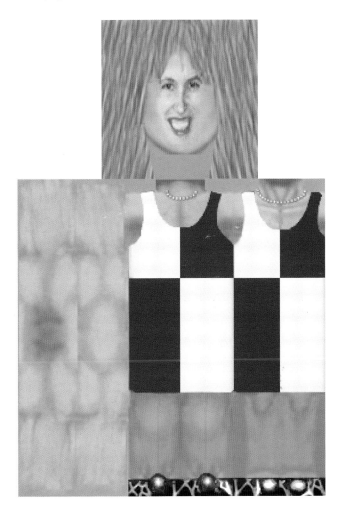

GAME SKINS, 2001

DESIGNERS
Mike Essl, b. 1975
Rob Reed, b. 1974
Matthew Richmond, b. 1974
The Chopping Block, Inc., New York

The "skins," or graphical personalities used in Web-based
games such as Quake and The Sims, are also known as
avatars. They are the digital surfaces of invented
personae. Below is a skin designed for the game Quake;
on the facing page are skins for The Sims game.

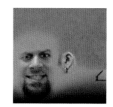

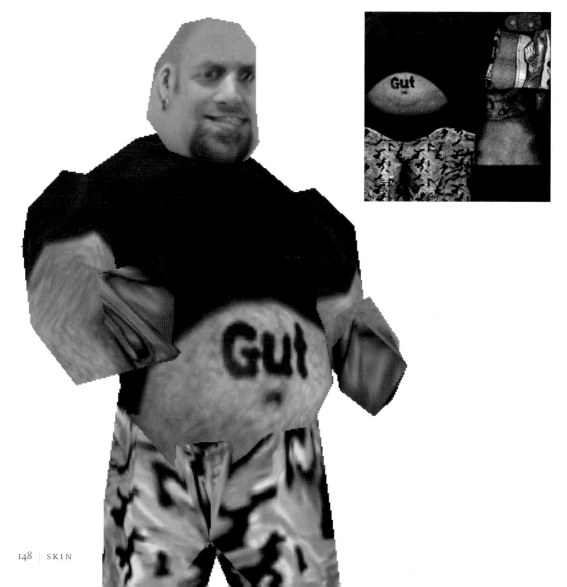

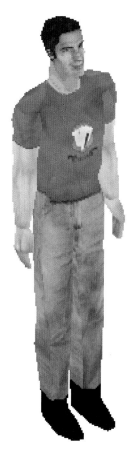

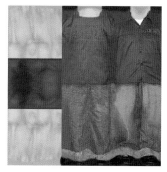
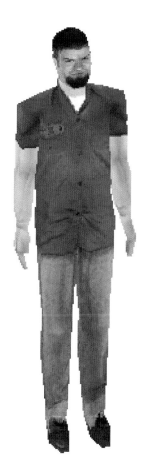
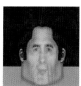
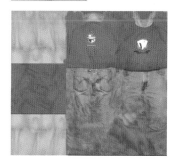

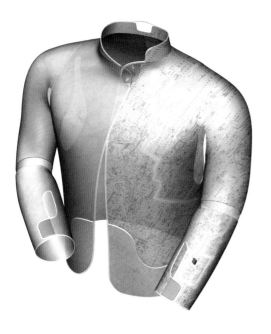

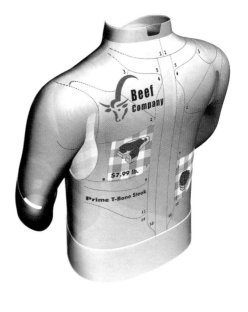

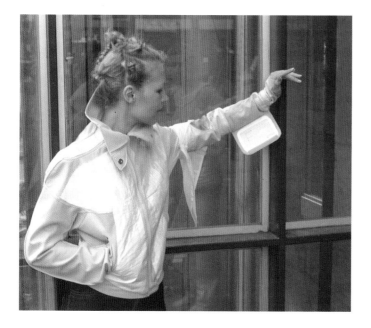

BLU, 2000, AND BLU2, 2001
Digital renderings and prototype
DESIGNERS Tad Toulis, b. 1967
Pierre-Yves DuBois, b. 1972
Lunar Design, Inc., San Francisco
TEAM Andrew Zee, Casey Wright,
Florence Bautista
PHOTOGRAPHY Sandbox Studio

These prototypes by Lunar Design explore
what could happen when digital displays
are thin, cheap, and flexible—when
electronically programmable paper comes
into its own as a material. Displays
composed of microscopic beads pick up
radio frequencies and then display specific
patterns. Shown above are two digital
renderings of BLU—a messenger's jacket
with a built-in global positioning system (GPS)
and an advertising surface. BLU2 (left) is a
physical prototype showing the integration
of hardware into the garment.

> *"TechnoLust seeks to merge the softness of skin with the hard lines of consumer electronics."*
> —Carla Murray and Peter Allen

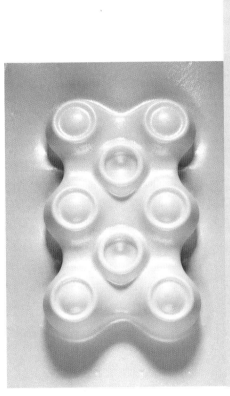

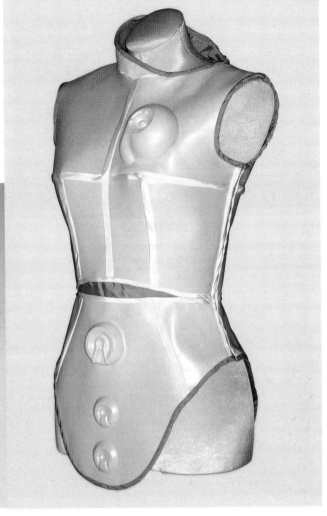

TECHNOLUST, 2000
Prototype for interactive garment

DESIGNERS   Carla Murray, b. 1970
Peter Allen, b. 1968
KnoWear, Cataumet, Massachusetts
Produced as graduate research at
Cranbrook Academy of Art, Michigan

PHOTOGRAPHY   Dan Forbes

TechnoLust is a prototype for a zip-on suit with integral electronic functions. Using 3d body scanning and vacuum forming processes, the suits would be manufactured on demand to fit individual needs, from body contours to technology preferences. Using such emerging technologies as nanochips, flexible printed circuitry, and soft screens, TechnoLust looks at the future of computing and communication technologies. The configuration of TechnoLust shown here—just one of many potential product variations— is a wireless, self-sufficient gaming suit, designed to allow the user to play virtual games from any location. The design is deliberately erotic, suggesting the replacement of erogenous zones with eletronic ports.

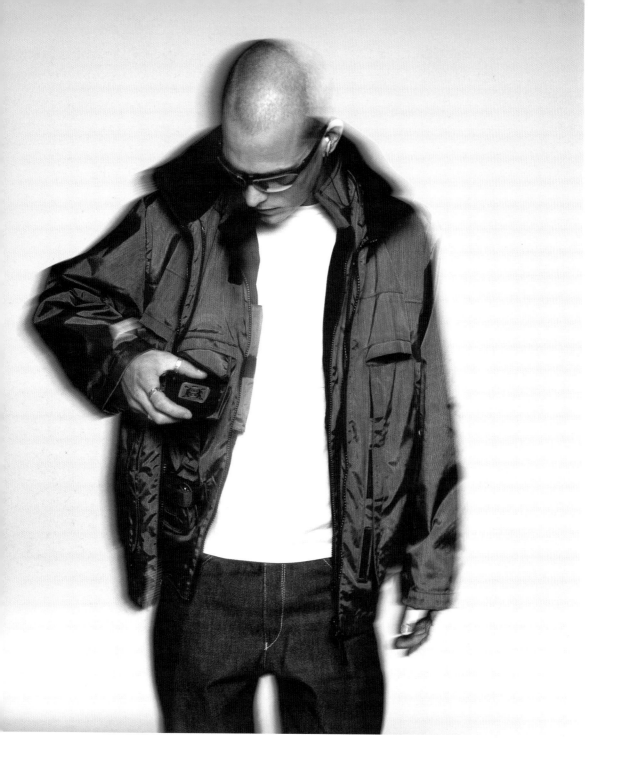

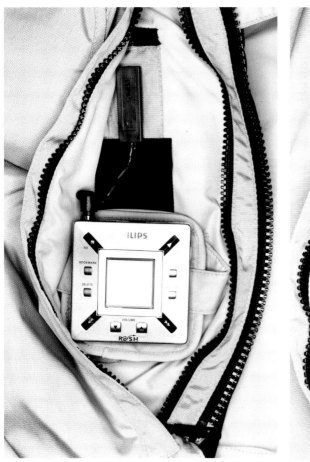
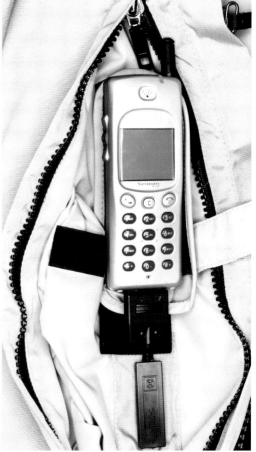

INDUSTRIAL CLOTHING LINE, 2000
Garment, metallic coated basket weave nylon,
rubber housings, wiring

DESIGNERS   Philips Design
               Massimo Osti, Levi's®

MANUFACTURER   Philips Electronics and Levi Strauss & Co.

PHOTOGRAPHY   Levi Strauss & Co.

The Industrial Clothing Line is a joint venture of Philips Electronics and Levi's. The jacket has a fully integrated communications and entertainment system. Philips earphones and a microphone are integrated into the collar. The earphones have an enlarged air chamber for enhanced sound, and users can switch between left only, right only, and stereo. When not in use the earphones can sit in rubber housing below the collar. A remote control links two originally separate hardware elements—a mobile phone and an MP3 player—thus enabling new functions, such as the downloading of music directly from the MP3 to the phone, the arrest of the MP3 function as soon as a call comes through the phone, or voice dial through a microphone inserted in the jacket collar.

"Increasingly, the digital realm penetrates and manifests itself through the physical realm of materials—unlike initial predictions, where the virtual was seen to be different from the physical."
—Sheila Kennedy

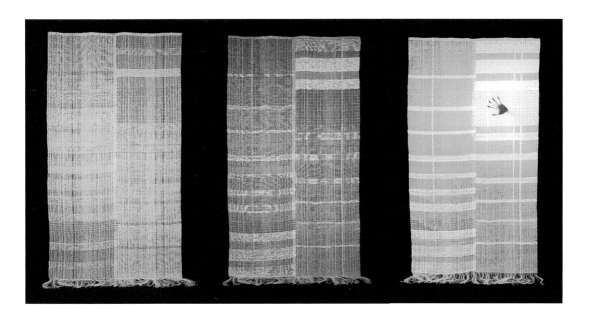

CHAMELEON CLOTH, GIVE BACK CURTAIN, 2001
Fabric, natural fiber blend woven with luminous phosphors
DESIGNER Sheila Kennedy, b. 1958
Kennedy & Violich Architecture, Boston
PROJECT ASSISTANT Dana Cho
Prototype commissioned by
Osram Opto-Semiconductors
Woven by Sheetal Khanna-Ravitch
PHOTOGRAPHY Doug Cogger

The Give Back Curtain is part of a series of surface designs by architect Sheila Kennedy that rethink the traditional and modern applications of the portable screen. The curtain is fabricated with photo-luminescent pigments in synthetic or natural fibers. Incidental light of a shorter wavelength, such as sunlight or fluorescent light, is absorbed by the fabric, retained, and then released as visible light. The light emission is designed as a dynamic light pattern that creates a series of color changes within the cloth. The curtain could be used to construct luminous enclosures that provide variable privacy, for use in residential, commercial, and workplace settings.

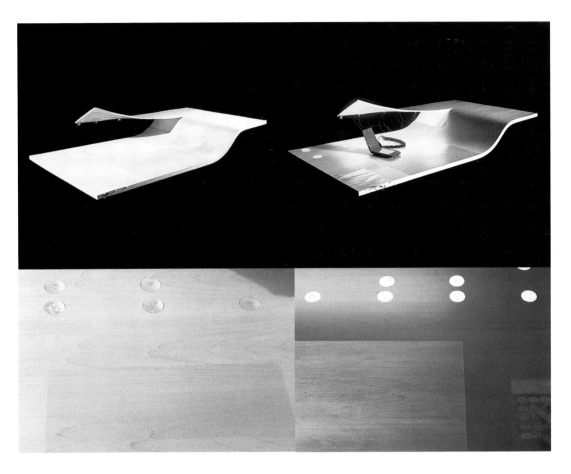

ELECTRIC PLYWOOD, 2000

Furniture, maple veneer plywood, electroluminescent film, integral digital tools

DESIGNER Sheila Kennedy
Kennedy & Violich Architecture, Boston

PROJECT ASSISTANT Veit Kugel

CARPENTRY Stephen Belton
EL film by Durel Corporation

(Clockwise, top left) *Inactive state, plywood desk top;*
Active state with handheld PDA appliance;
Surface detail, wood with Memory Blotter, inactive state;
Surface detail, activated Memory Blotter, embedded
data ports, and calculator

The Electric Plywood Desk is an energy efficient, interactive wood surface. Ultra-thin polymer films are layered between the plywood laminations. The films conduct electricity, information, and electro-luminescent (EL) light. Digital fabrication techniques are used to form the plywood so that light washes across its surface. This illumination charges a Memory Blotter that has been impregnated with a luminous phosphor which then absorbs and recycles the light. When the EL light is turned off, the Memory Blotter glows, providing an independent source of light. Handheld PDAs can be plugged into ports integrated into the wood surface. Digital tools can be embedded into the desk, where they are activated by touch via a springy, resilient wood veneer.

CHROMAZONE, 1999
Table, heat sensitive polymer,
and steel square tubing
DESIGNER   Karim Rashid, b. 1960
Karim Rashid, Inc., New York
MANUFACTURER   Totem, New York

This table by Karim Rashid has a surface that changes color in response to heat. The tabletop becomes a visual index of the rituals and interactions performed on it, from elbows and hands leaning on the surface to hot cups and dishes.

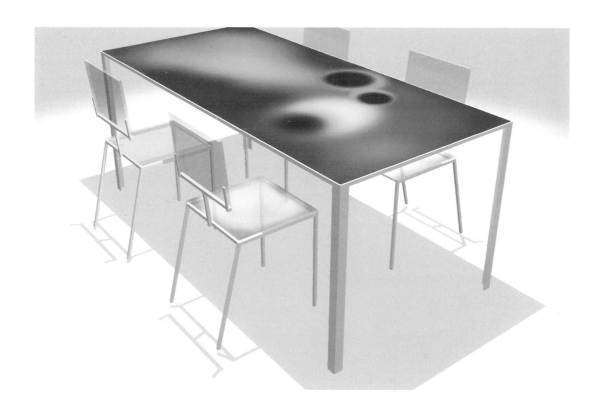

MN02 BONANZA, 2000
Bicycle, aluminum, photoluminescent paint,
and other materials
DESIGNER   Marc Newson, b. 1963
Marc Newson Ltd., United Kingdom
MANUFACTURER   Biomega, Denmark
PHOTOGRAPHY   Tue Schioerring

The body of this bicycle designed by Marc Newson has a
membranelike connecting structure. The frame is coated in
tritrium, a photoluminescent paint that provides a beautiful
and traffic-safe glow in the dark.

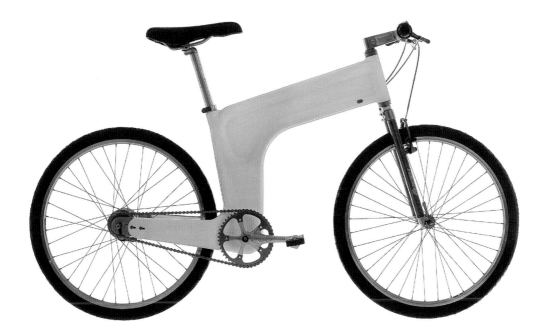

artificial light
+
artificial life

SKIN is said to "glow" in response to youth, health, or happiness. Yet few creatures actually emit light from their bodies.

A glowing object appears curiously alive. Countless products, from televisions and desktop computers to phones, handheld games, and personal assistants, communicate through glowing screens. Artificial light signals the presence of electricity, the energy that animates the object world. Electrical current is cyborg blood, the life force of digital and mechanical systems.

While some lighting systems serve to illuminate an object, environment, or task area, others emit low levels of light to foreground the lighting fixture itself. Light emanates from soft, heavy blobs of gel or from bulbs festooned with silicone growths. Ordinary domestic goods—blankets, pillows, or chairs—come alive as they glow with artificial light. While most fixtures must be shielded from touch, these objects invite physical contact. Their dull interior illumination draws attention to the surface, infusing their skins with an alien energy, at once comforting and strange.

"BUT THE FEMALE WAS DRAWN
TO SOMETHING FAR MORE GENTLE
IN THE MALE," 2000
Photograph

PHOTOGRAPHY Elinor Carucci, b. 1971
COURTESY OF Ricco/Maresca Gallery, New York

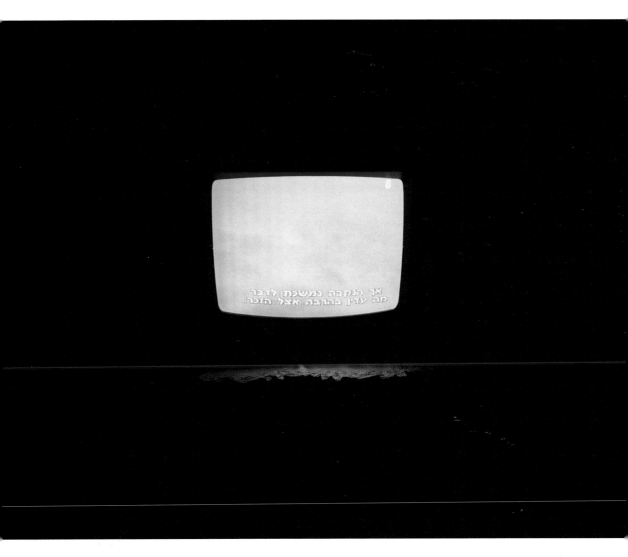

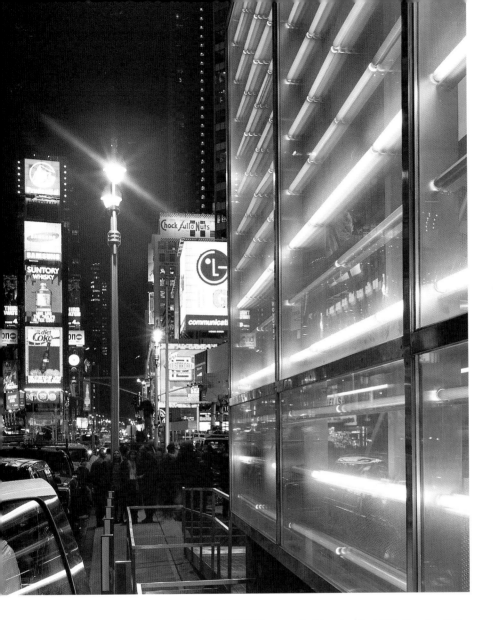

U.S. ARMED FORCES RECRUITING
STATION, TIMES SQUARE, NEW YORK
1999

DESIGNERS Stephen Cassell, b. 1963
Adam Yarinsky, b. 1962
ARO (Architecture Research Office), New York

PROJECT ARCHITECT Alan Bruton

TEAM Heather Roberge, Scott Abrahams,
Eric Ajemian

PHOTOGRAPHY David Joseph

Each long facade of ARO's Recruiting Station
for the U.S. Armed Forces is an American
flag made of thirteen bands of fluorescent
tubing. Translucent reflective gels create
colored light at night while reflecting natural
light by day. The flags are integrated into a
custom stainless steel and glass window
wall, so that the flag lights are layered with
reflections of the surrounding streetscape.
The building varies between reflectivity and
transparency, depending on ambient lighting
conditions and the position of the viewer.

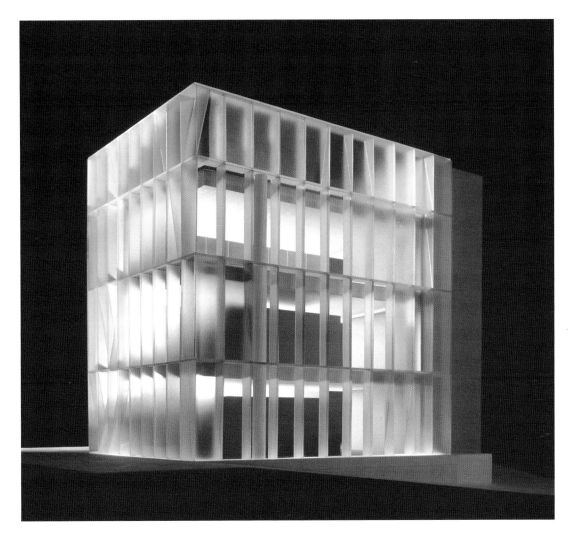

HELMUT LANG TOKYO, 2001
Architectural model, MDF, chipboard, acrylic
Digital rendering
DESIGNERS Richard Gluckman, b. 1947
Melissa Cicetti, b. 1967
Brett Tipert, b. 1967
Gluckman Mayner Architects, New York
TEAM Alex Stoltz, Julie Torres Moskovitz,
Sarah Ludington
PHOTOGRAPHY Jock Pottle © Esto

The facade of the Helmut Lang Tokyo showroom, designed by Gluckman Mayner Architects, is composed of translucent glass and LCD glass panels. Sixty centimeters deep, the facade is a vast showcase and a field of dynamic light patterns, shifting from opaque to transparent to translucent over the course of the day. The variations in the facade either reveal or conceal the content inside the building: the merchandise, the customers, or simply the concrete shell within.

BOALUM, 1969

Flexible lamp, PVC plastic, metal

DESIGNERS Livio Castiglioni, 1911–1979

Gianfranco Frattini, b. 1926

MANUFACTURER Artemide, Italy

COLLECTION OF Cooper-Hewitt, National Design Museum,

Smithsonian Institution, The Decorative Arts

Association Acquisitions Fund, 1991-47-8

PHOTOGRAPHY Matt Flynn

Designed in the Pop ethos of antiformality, the Boalum lamp rejects the vertical symmetry of traditional lighting fixtures in favor of a flexible, malleable form with no base. The Baolum can be draped over and around furniture, or it can rest on the floor, coiled up like a glowing primordial worm.

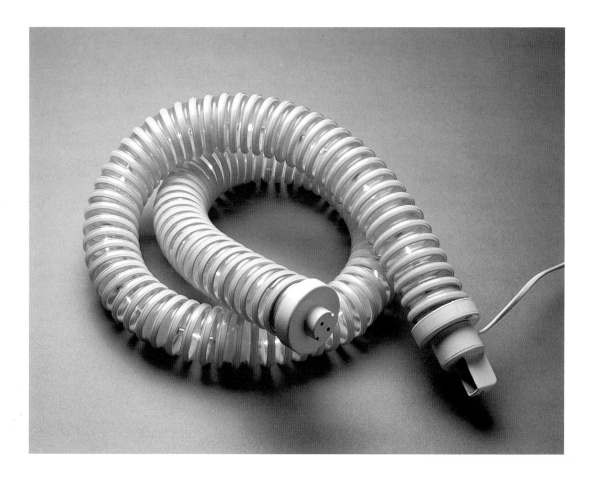

GLOBJECT, 1999

Lighting fixture, limited edition of five

Two electroluminescent sheets (one facing up,
one down), soft polyurethane resin, cables

DESIGNER Karim Rashid, b. 1960

MANUFACTURER Trans>6, U.S.A.

Karim Rashid's soft, glowing blob is tumescent
with alien life. Resting heavily on a table or floor,
it resembles a primitive organism waiting
to evolve.

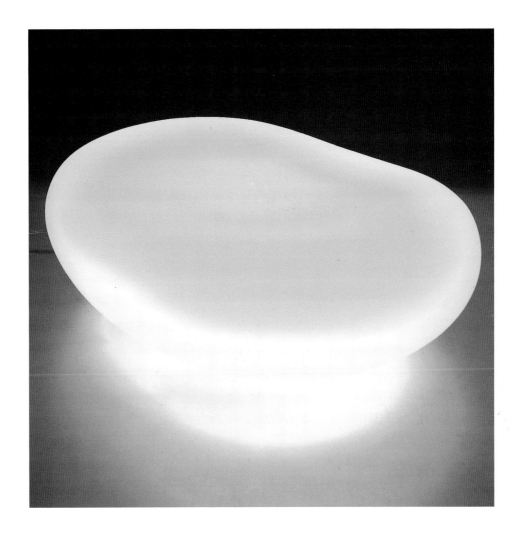

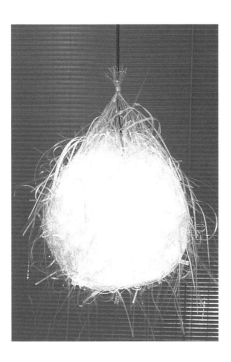

TOP SECRET, 2000

Lighting fixture, polyester film, compact fluorescent light, nylon net
DESIGNER Héctor Serrano, b. 1974
MANUFACTURER Héctor Serrano, United Kingdom
PHOTOGRAPHY Jordi Adriá

This lamp by Hector Serrano is made from acetate that has been passed through a shredding machine. The acetate strips are held together with a clear nylon net, like that used for packing oranges. The result is a semitransparent cocoon of irregularly massed material.

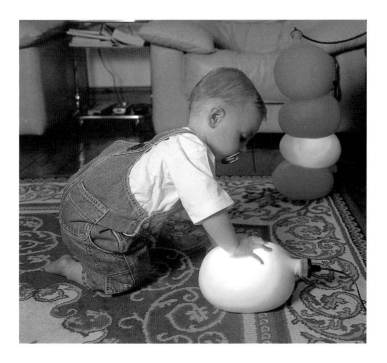

SUPER PATATA, 2000

Lighting, latex, salt, compact fluorescent light
DESIGNER
Héctor Serrano, b. 1974
MANUFACTURER
DMD, The Netherlands
Droog Design Collection
PHOTOGRAPHY Jordi Adriá

Hector Serrano's Super Patata is a salt-filled latex bladder with a fluorescent bulb at its core. This touchable lamp can be used as a pillow, antistress device, or bedwarmer, as well as for direct or ambient illumination. The lamps can be stacked, mounding like nesting creatures.

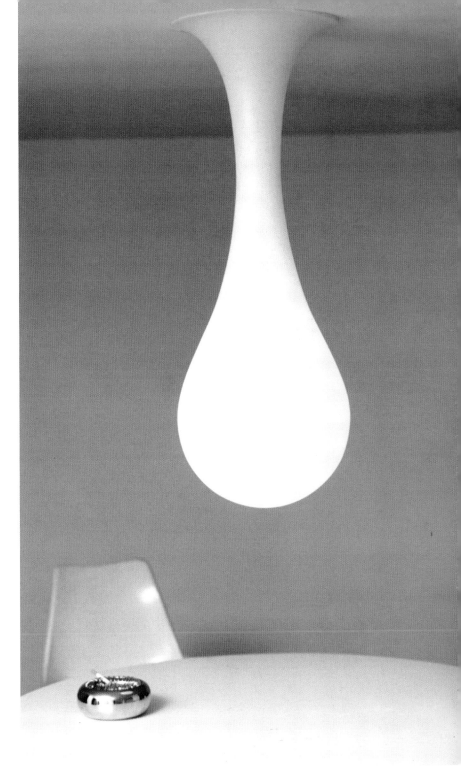

LIQUID_LIGHT: DROP_1
1999
Lighting fixture, plastic,
hardware
DESIGNERS
Constantin Wortmann, b. 1970
Benjamin Hopf, b. 1971
Büro für Form, Munich
MANUFACTURER
Next, Germany
PHOTOGRAPHY David Steets

This ceiling lamp, from a series
of four fixtures designed by
Constantin Wortmann and
Benjamin Hopf, appears to
ooze from above.

BUBBLE, 2000

Soft silicone light, powered by LEDs and rechargeable batteries, with charger and bubble love included

DESIGNERS Aaron Rincover, b. 1970
Mathmos Design Team

MANUFACTURER Mathmos, United Kingdom

PHOTOGRAPHY Vanessa Stump

Aaron Rincover's soft, ball-shaped, battery-operated lights are turned on by a squeeze of the hand. Rejecting the standard conception of the electrical fixture that is tied to a specific domestic tableau, these portable units provide illumination for the nomadic life.

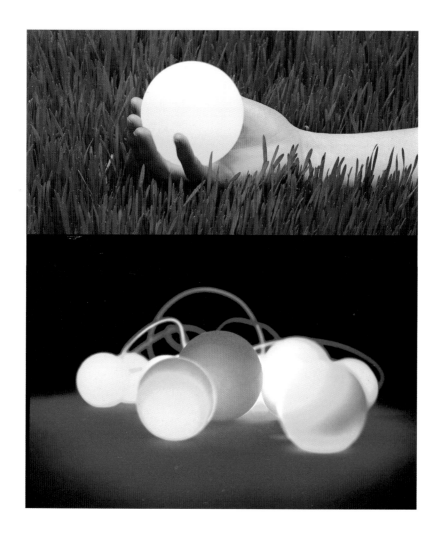

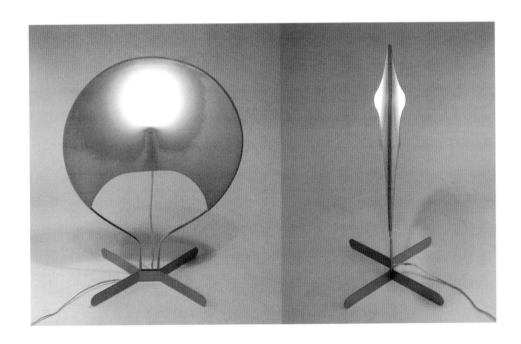

PALOMBELLA, 2000

Lighting fixture, steel, silicone rubber cap,
lightbulbs

DESIGNER Paolo Ulian, b. 1961

MANUFACTURER Floetotto, Germany

PHOTOGRAPHY Paolo Ulian

Paolo Ulian's Palombella lamp is made from four
simple elements that can be easily assembled
and disassembled. A silicone rubber bathing cap
is stretched across a steel-rod frame. The energy-
saving lightbulb presses through the rubber
membrane, swelling its flat surface.

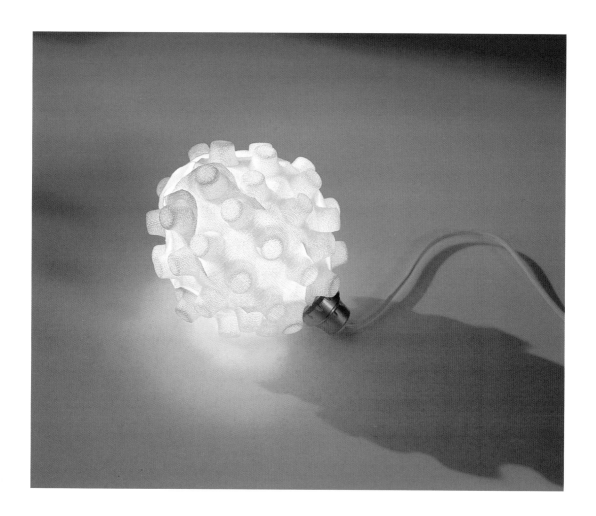

WOO ORB, 2000
Lighting fixture, 3d mesh textile and
lighting hardware
DESIGNERS Don Carr, b. 1959
Aaron Double, b. 1975
TEAM Liza Lamb, Emma Jones
MANUFACTURER Woo, U.S.A.
PHOTOGRAPHY Tom Wedell

The shade of Don Carr's Woo Orb
is made from a molded 3d fabric.
The lamp can rest on a table or
hang from the ceiling, singly or in
groups.

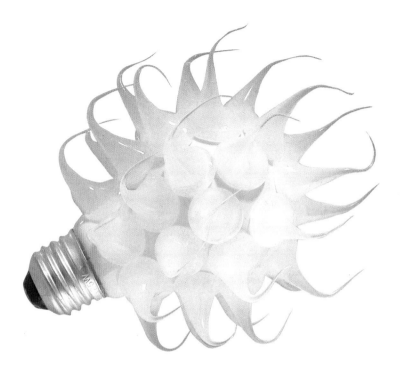

UBO LITE, 1998
Silicone, standard lightbulb
DESIGNERS Uri Ben-Or, b. 1970
Yuval Dor, b. 1968
MANUFACTURER MeWe International/Kikkerland
Design, Inc., New York
Ubo Lite first shown and produced
by Yuval Design Studio Gallery,
Tel Aviv, 1998

Created by Israeli designer Uri Ben-Or, the Ubo Lite is a standard bulb encrusted with growthlike dollops of silicone. The bulbs are sold in Urban Outfitters stores in the United States, a venue purveying fashion and housewears to the teen and young adult market. The bulbs can be used in common light fixtures, instantly transforming an ordinary lamp into an alien artifact.

RUBBER LAMP NO. 5, 2000

Prototype, silicone, wiring, electric lamp

DESIGNERS   Robert Moorhead, b. 1972
              Granger Moorhead, b. 1969
              Moorhead & Moorhead
              Bill Stewart of Sculpture City, Inc.

PHOTOGRAPHY   Robert Moorhead

This lamp by architects and industrial designers Robert and Granger Moorhead consists of a flexible silicone shell that flips up or down to provide either ambient or task lighting. The glowing rubber flesh resembles a pod or cocoon harboring alien life.

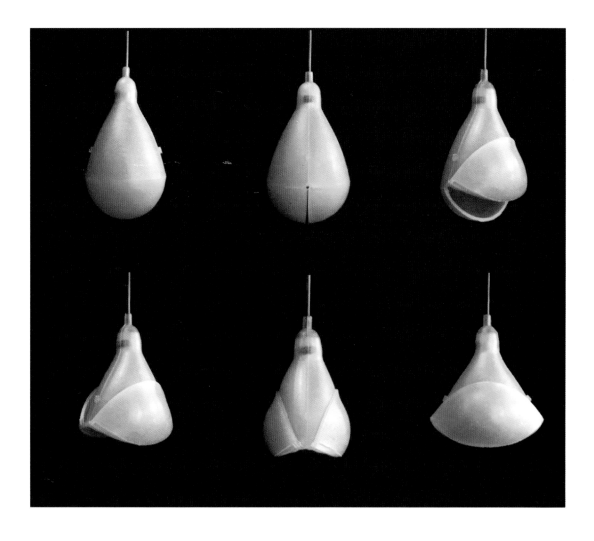

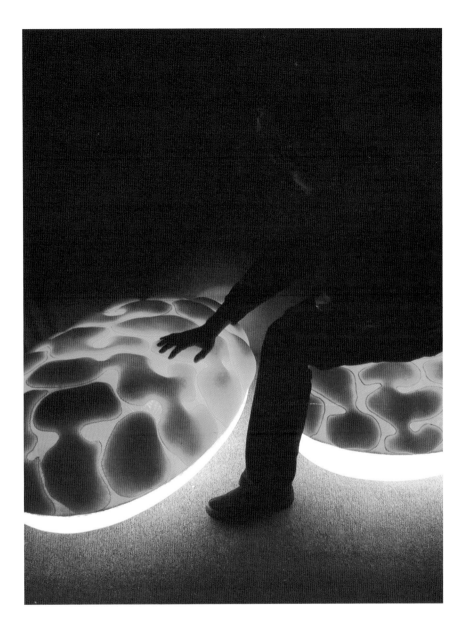

LIGHTSEAT, 2000
Lycra fabric cover with polypropylene grain,
polyester resin seat with TL light

DESIGNER Eelco van der Meer, b. 1973
MANUFACTURER Eelco van der Meer, Velp, Netherlands
PHOTOGRAPHY Eelco van der Meer

Eelco van der Meer refers to his Lightseat—a glowing
piece of furniture that provides both seating and
illumination—as "lightcandy for the mind." Its top is
covered with an overscaled reptilian skin of quilted fabric,
while its bottom glows naked white. Evoking the merging
of egg and organism, this object is a hypertrophic ode
to artificial light and artificial life.

THE PILLOW, 1999
Lighting fixture, cotton, organza,
plastic, lightbulb
DESIGNER   Sanne Lund Traberg, b. 1971
MANUFACTURER   Frandsen Lyskilde, Denmark
PHOTOGRAPHY   Sanne Lund Traberg

Sanne Lund Traberg's pillow light is stuffed
with organza, cushioning an electric bulb
at its interior. The cotton pillowcase can be
removed for washing. A long cord allows
the object to be freely moved about.

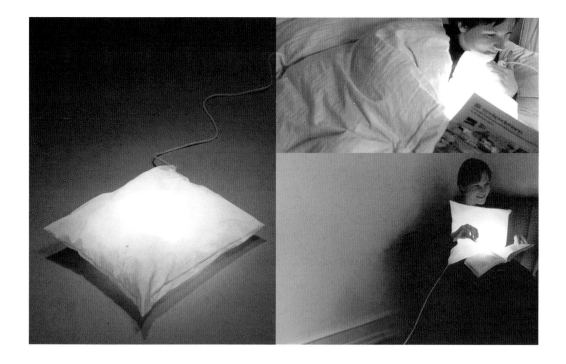

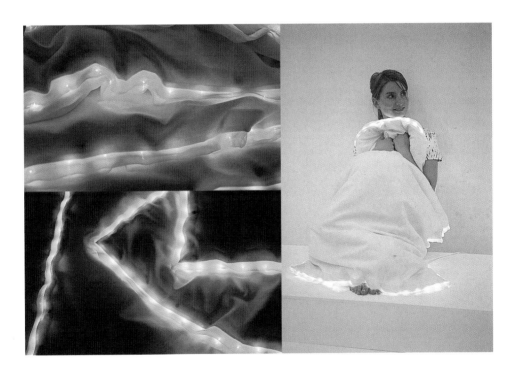

BLANKET, 2000
Prototype lighting fixture, wool, silk, cotton,
lightbulbs

DESIGNER Ditte Hammerstroem, b. 1971

PHOTOGRAPHY Ditte Hammerstroem

Ditte Hammerstroem's illuminated blanket transforms
an ordinary object of domestic comfort into a
responsive organism. The edge of the blanket is
bordered with tiny lightbulbs, providing illumination for
reading in bed or in an armchair. The border lights up
when touched. The outerlayer of the blanket is wool
and can be removed and washed.

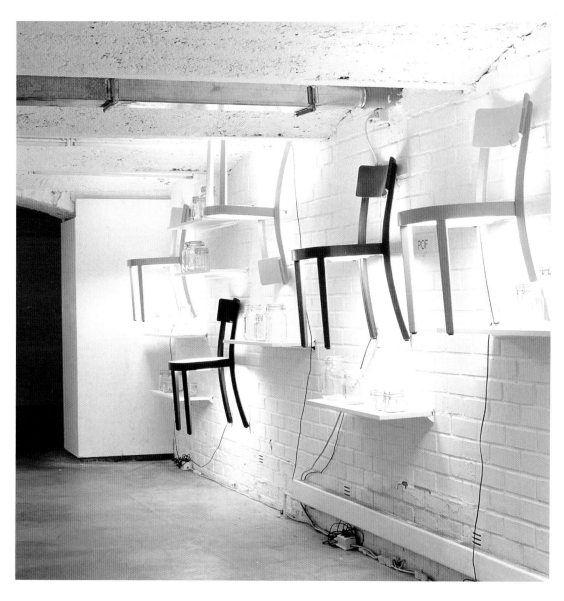

POF 1, 2000

Lighting and seating, beech wood, Lexan,
fluorescent lamp

DESIGNERS   Horgen-Glarus and N2, Switzerland

MANUFACTURER   hidden®, The Netherlands

PHOTOGRAPHY   Wouter

The Swiss company Horgen-Glarus has been producing this classic
wooden chair since 1916. The Swiss design firm N2 updated the chair
by illuminating its seat. Made from a sheet of translucent plastic, the
new base contains a fluorescent bulb.

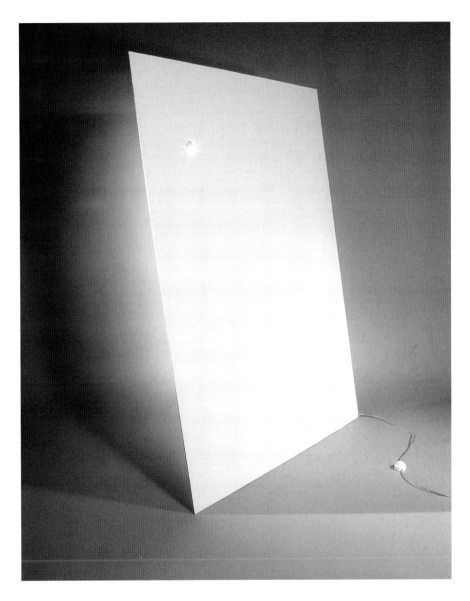

WHAT A LITTLE MOONLIGHT
CAN DO, 1998
Lighting, Alucobond,
halogen lamp
DESIGNER   Kazuhiro Yamanaka, b. 1971
MANUFACTURER   Boffi, Italy
PHOTOGRAPHY   Philip Vile

Kazuhiro Yamanaka's planar light fixture consists of a halogen lamp mounted at the edge of a hole in a sheet of Alucobond, a layer of plastic sandwiched between two layers of aluminum. The metal surfaces conduct electricity, lighting the halogen lamp without wires. When the sheet leans against a wall, light is emitted between the wall and the sheet, creating a serene glow.

padding
+
protection

SKIN has a complex and vital interior beneath its dead outer surface. Skin's middle layer, the dermis, is a dense substance made of collagen and elastic fibers, while the innermost layer of fat insulates heat and protects against injury. These hidden layers provide the supportive padding that shapes the body's outer envelope.

The international Pop movement that burst forth in the 1960s explored the possibilities of inflatable forms—plastic skins pumped with air. Such artifacts subverted values of permanence in favor of lightness, portability, and disposability. In a similar spirit, Pop designers made objects out of synthetic foams, eliminating the heavy internal armature of wood or metal in favor of creating objects that are all flesh. These ideas have been revived and expanded over the past decade, as designers have explored new forms and materials.

Clothing supplements the skin's defenses against the elements. Contemporary designers have hyper-extended fashion's protective capacity, creating garments that serve as portable environments for the modern nomad, set loose in a wilderness defined by work and leisure as well as the forces of nature.

ZIPPER MARK, 1999
Photograph
PHOTOGRAPHY   Elinor Carucci, b. 1971
COURTESY OF   Ricco/Maresca Gallery, New York

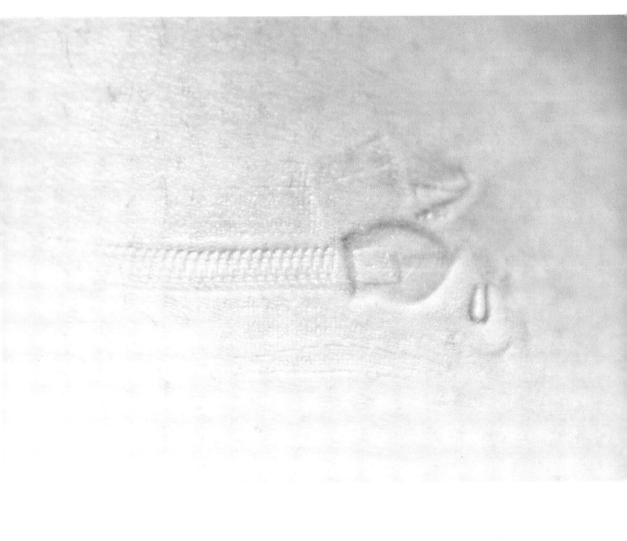

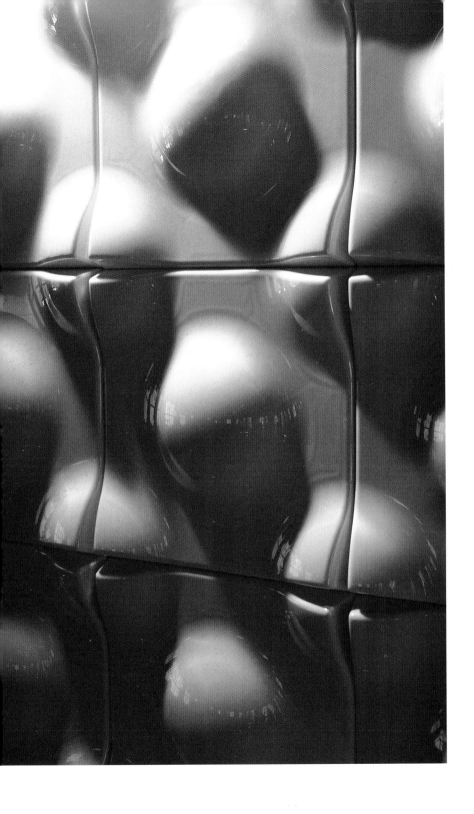

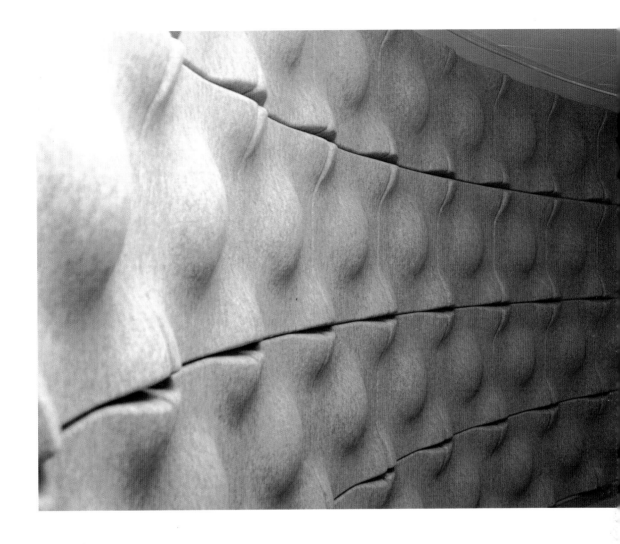

SOUNDWAVE SWELL, 1999–2000
Acoustic panels, plastic, molded
polyester fiber

DESIGNER Teppo Asikainen, b. 1968

MANUFACTURER Snowcrash, Sweden

PHOTOGRAPHY Snowcrash

Soundwave is a series of acoustical panels used to absorb
and diffuse sound in noisy interiors. Swell (above) is made
of molded polyester fibers, built up into a thick, dimensional,
synthetic felt. Swell Diffuser (left) is a hard plastic surface,
enhancing acoustic control by diffusing sound.

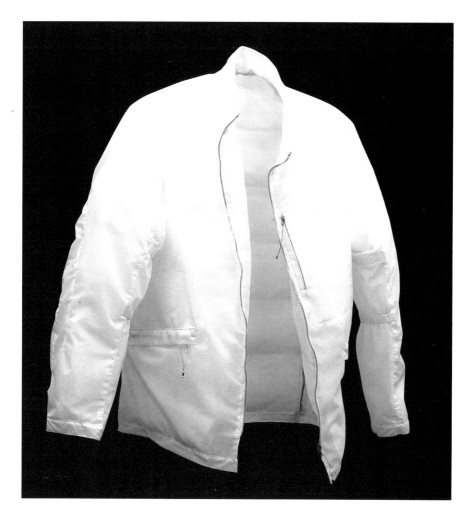

ABSOLUTE ZERO, 1999

Garment, Aerogel, fabric, PET

DESIGNER Mauro Taliani, b. 1958

MANUFACTURER Corpo Nove, Italy

Aerogel supplied by Marketech International,
Port Townsend, Washington

PHOTOGRAPHY Alberto Petra

Aerogel is one of the lightest substances on earth; it is also an excellent insulator, making it an appropriate material for expeditions—to outer space or the Arctic Circle—requiring lightweight protection from the elements. Invented in the 1930s, Aerogel was used to insulate the Mars Pathfinder in 1999. To create this hyperinsulated jacket, the Italian sportswear company Corpo Nove sewed bags of powdered Aerogel between two layers of fabric, creating an extremely warm, light coat.

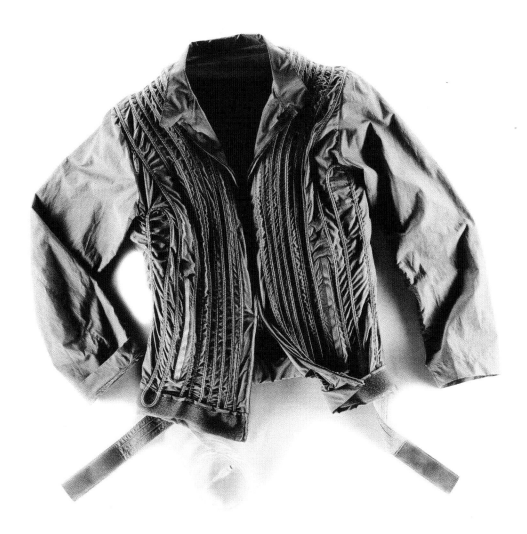

COOLING SYSTEM, 1999

Garment, nylon, leather, plastic tubing

DESIGNER Mauro Taliani

MANUFACTURER Corpo Nove, Italy

Original cooling system developed and commercialized by DTI-Delta Temax Inc., Canada

PHOTOGRAPHY Alberto Petra

This jacket is based on a miniaturized air-conditioning system that was commissioned by the U.S. Army during the Cold War. It was designed to be fitted to the inside of combat clothing, allowing soldiers to fight and survive in conditions of extreme heat—perhaps after a nuclear blast. A similar system is used for cooling astronaut's suits. Fifty meters of 2-millimeter-wide plastic tubing are needed to constuct the internal cooling circuit in Corpo Nove's Cooling System jacket.

ORICALCO, 2001

Garment, Memory Metal (fabric made from
50% titanium and mix of other alloys)

DESIGNER Mauro Taliani, b. 1958

MANUFACTURER Corpo Nove, Bacagli, and Texteam, Italy

PHOTOGRAPHY Alberto Petra

This men's shirt by Corpo Nove is woven with titanium, which
allows the fabric to react to temperature shifts. The shirt holds its
wrinkles when bunched up, and then instantly relaxes when
exposed to a current of hot air (as from an electric hair dryer).
The shirt can thus be "ironed" while its user wears it, and creases
and 3d elements can be embedded in the fabric's memory.

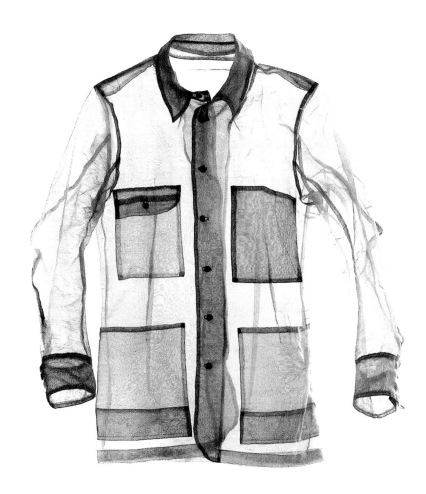

Y WAY, 2001
Windbreaker, Teflon-coated cashmere
DESIGNER Yves Béhar, b. 1967
fuseproject, San Francisco
CREATIVE DIRECTORS Tina Lutz and Marcia Patmos
Lutz & Patmos, New York
Made in Italy
PHOTOGRAPHY Bert Spangemacher

Yves Béhar has updated a traditional, luxurious, natural material—cashmere—by coating it with Teflon. The water-repellant windbreaker was commissioned by Lutz & Patmos, maker of cashmere garments and accessories in a modern idiom.

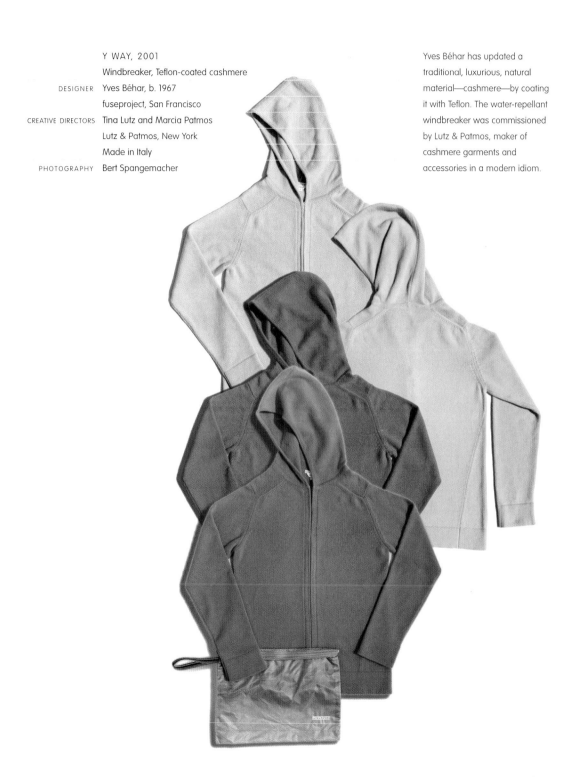

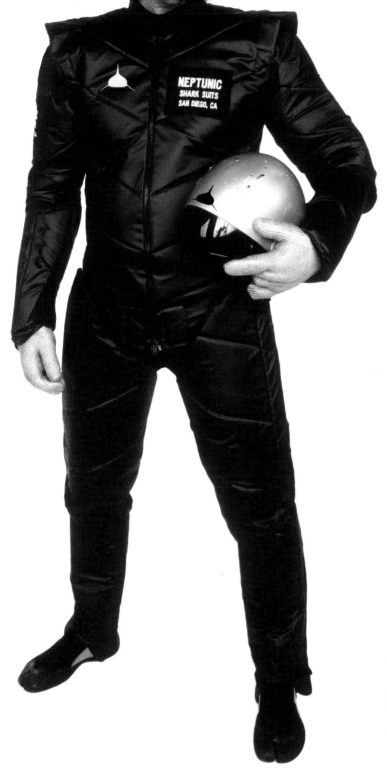

NEPTUNIC SHARK SUIT:
NEMO II, 2001
Protective garment
Vectran (liquid crystal polymer fiber),
steel mesh, carbon fiber laminate
DESIGNERS Jeremiah Sullivan, b. 1954
Kym Milburn, b. 1962
MANUFACTURER Neptunic Shark Suits,
San Diego, California
Steel mesh fabricated by
Azon Corporation

Jeremiah Sullivan pioneered the steel
mesh shark suit in the early 1980s to
enable researchers and enthusiasts to
swim with sharks. The new Nemo II is
made of a proprietary fabric that is
lightweight and bite-resistant. The suit
is worn with a submersible helmet and
steel mesh gloves and socks. The
Nemo II offers substantial protection
against shark attacks: "Interaction with
nature's predators can be dangerous
business, and no suit can protect a fool
from himself. The shark suit was
designed to provide man with the
opportunity to more safely interact with
the sea and all its spectacular
inhabitants."

SPEEDO® FASTSKIN™, 1999
Garment, nylon and Lycra textured
with v-shaped ridge pattern based
on sharkskin

MANUFACTURER SPEEDO®, a division
of The Warnaco Group, Inc.

PHOTOGRAPHY Mark Weiss

The SPEEDO Fastskin swimsuit created
an international sensation during
the 2000 Olympics, when it helped
swimmers improve their times by
decreasing drag and turbulence. The
suit's surface is based on sharkskin,
whose dermal denticles—which look
like tiny hydrofoils with V-shaped
ridges—direct the flow of water over
the shark's body. The Fastskin fabric
duplicates the height, width, and exact
proportion of the shark's dermal
denticles. The super-stretch fabric
retains its shape and compresses the
swimmer's muscles, reducing muscle
vibration and thus lessening fatigue.
A special gripper fabric on the forearm
of the suit mimics the swimmer's
natural skin, enhancing "sensory
feedback."

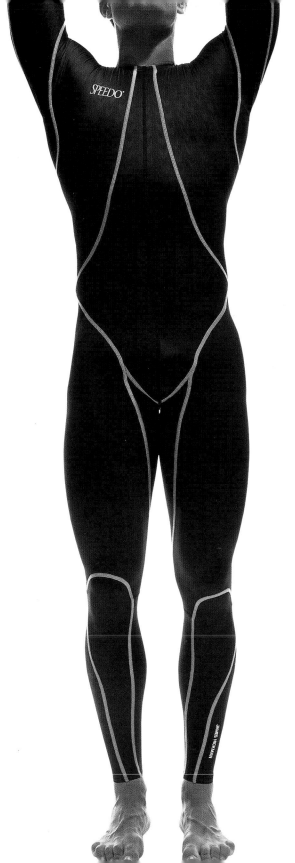

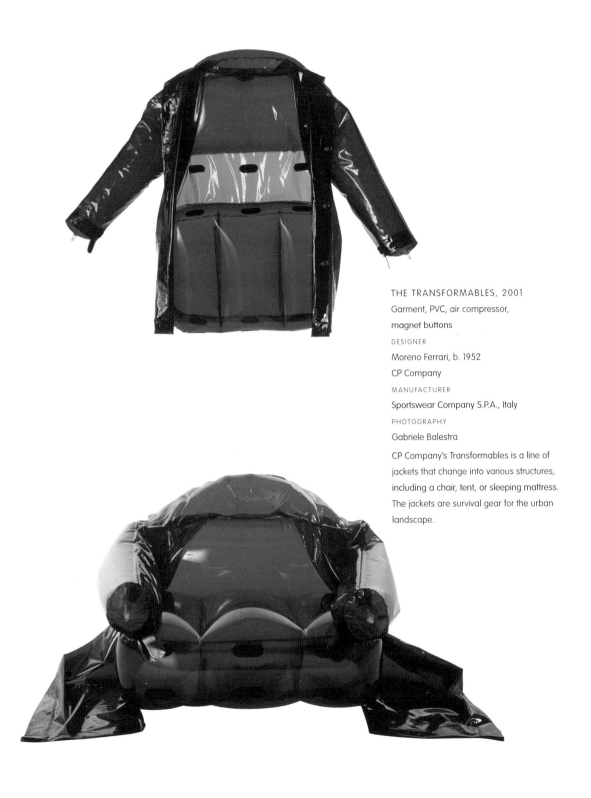

THE TRANSFORMABLES, 2001
Garment, PVC, air compressor,
magnet buttons
DESIGNER
Moreno Ferrari, b. 1952
CP Company
MANUFACTURER
Sportswear Company S.P.A., Italy
PHOTOGRAPHY
Gabriele Balestra

CP Company's Transformables is a line of
jackets that change into various structures,
including a chair, tent, or sleeping mattress.
The jackets are survival gear for the urban
landscape.

VINYL SUIT, 1998

DESIGNER

Walter van Beirendonck, b. 1957
W&LT (Wild and Lethal Trash), Belgium
Collection of Walter van Beirendonck

PHOTOGRAPHY Dan Lecca

Walter van Beirendonck was an original
member of the Antwerp Six, a group of
fashion designers coming out of the Academy
of Fine Arts, Antwerp, in the early 1980s.
Whereas many of his Belgian contemporaries
are known to use natural materials in
somber, neutral tones, Beirendonck employs
synthetic fabrics in harsh colors. Here, a shiny
red suit is covered with hard, plastic *pastilles,*
suggesting the scales of a fantastic dragon.
According to Beirendonck, the surface is
designed to protect and amaze. "The body of
the future," he says, "will be different."

KILLER, 1996

Jacket, vinyl

DESIGNER Walter van Beirendonck

MANUFACTURER W&LT (Wild and Lethal Trash), Belgium

PHOTOGRAPHY Chris Ruggie

This pink vinyl jacket has nozzles for inflating, like those on a
pool toy. The jacket is designed to reshape the body—in place
of vigorous workouts, simply blow up your muscles.

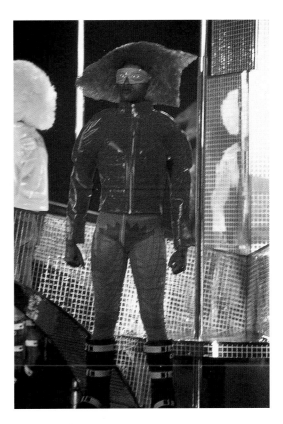

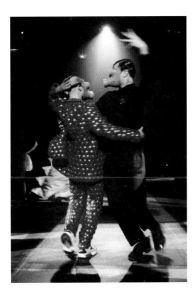

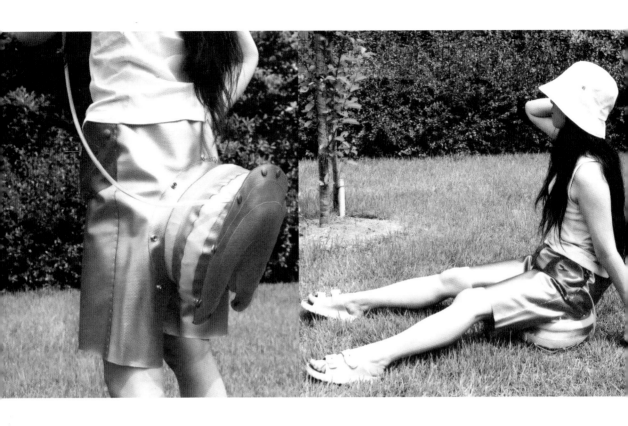

HOMEWEAR STOOLPANTS, 2001
Garment, inflatable PVC, plastic tubing

DESIGNERS   Izumi Kohama, b. 1968
Xavier Moulin, b. 1969
ixilab, Japan

Stoolpants is a pair of translucent plastic shorts
fitted with a cushion in the rear. The user inflates
the stool by blowing into a plastic tube. Stoolpants
is part of the Homewear line, created by Izumi
Kohama and Xavier Moulin, partners in ixilab.
Looking at contemporary nomadic living,
Homewear addresses the need for personal
equipment that provides rest and refuge in public
places, offering tiny points of escape from the
overwhelming stimuli of work and leisure.

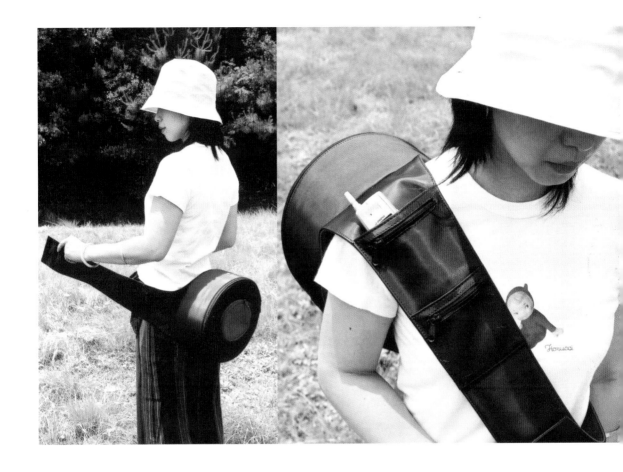

HOMEWEAR PUFYBAG, 2001
Garment, cordura and nylon fabrics, PVC
inflatable ring, plastic zippers, Velcro

DESIGNERS Izumi Kohama
Xavier Moulin
ixilab, Japan

Pufybag is worn over the shoulder like a backpack. A Velcro
fastening allows the user to adjust its size. Objects can be stored
inside the bag, which has a PVC inflatable ring around the main
pocket. The bag thus serves as a portable stool as well as a
container.

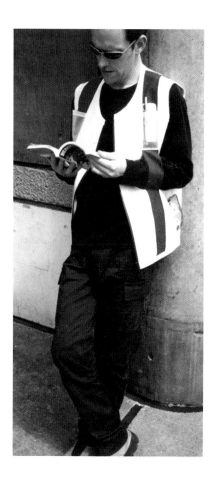

PACK CHAIR, 2000
Prototype, polyester cloth and
netting, polyurethane foam
DESIGNER
François Azambourg, b. 1963
MANUFACTURER
V.I.A. (prototype), France
Appel Permanent V.I.A. 2000
PHOTOGRAPHY   Samuel Gomez

Turn the knob on François
Azambourg's Pack, and a
compressed mass of fabric and
netting fills up with material to
become a rigid chair. The knob
releases two liquid components
that chemically react and expand
to fill their fabric skin.

HOMEWEAR MANGASTRAP, 2001
Garment, cordura and nylon fabrics, foam
rubber, plastic zippers, Velcro
DESIGNERS
Izumi Kohama
Xavier Moulin
ixilab, Japan

Mangastrap is designed for readers of mangas
(Japanese comic books). This gear supports the
wearer's arms, allow him or her to stand and
read comfortably. It is a skin that prevents fatigue
by holding up the skeleton.

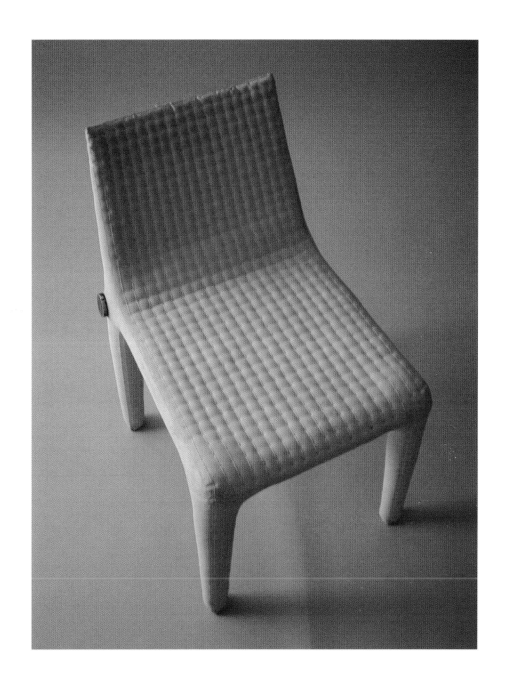

GLOBULO, 1999
Pouf, PVC
DESIGNERS   Fabrizio Bertero, b. 1965
             Andrea Panto, b. 1974
MANUFACTURER Zanotta, Italy
PHOTOGRAPHY Marino Ramazzotti

The Italian manufacturer Zanotta introduced some of the first mass-produced inflatable furniture in the late 1960s. Zanotta recently issued its own contribution to the revival of 1960s Pop design: Globulo, a series of inflatable chairs resembling bright translucent candies. These invertebrate objects conflate structure and skin. Air becomes a physical material, given form by the surrounding membrane.

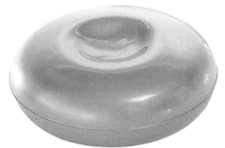

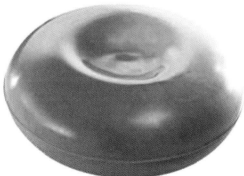

SPHERIZE AND COOLER, 2000

Furniture, polyethylene

DESIGNERS Valerie Kiock, b. 1971
Kuno Nüssli, b. 1970
N2, Switzerland

MANUFACTURER hidden®, Netherlands

PHOTOGRAPHY Wouter

Spherize (by Valerie Kiock) and Cooler (by Kiock and Kuno Nüssli), are an inflatable table and chair. Cooler has a hole in the top for keeping a bottle chilled. Both are outfitted with a valve allowing the user to adjust the pressure to suit his or her preference for firmer or softer seating. The furniture inflates with a bicycle pump. Drawing on Pop sensibilities, these pieces assume crisper, more geometric lines.

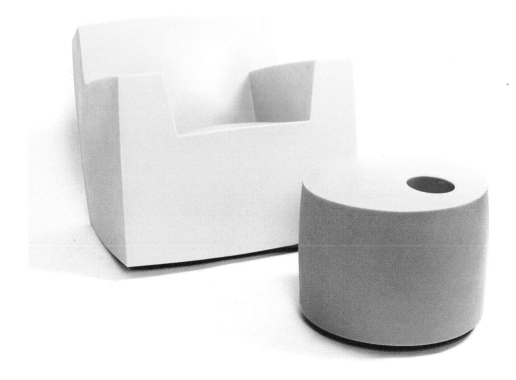

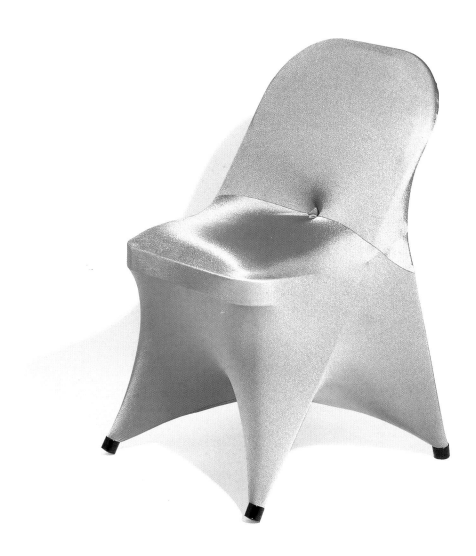

CHAIR COCOON, 1999
Slipcover, stretch fabric
DESIGNER
Anne Masako Moss, b. 1960
MANUFACTURER
Masacco New York
PHOTOGRAPHY   Mark Viker

Anne Masako Moss's inexpensive slipcover creates a taut,
elastic skin around a standard metal folding chair.

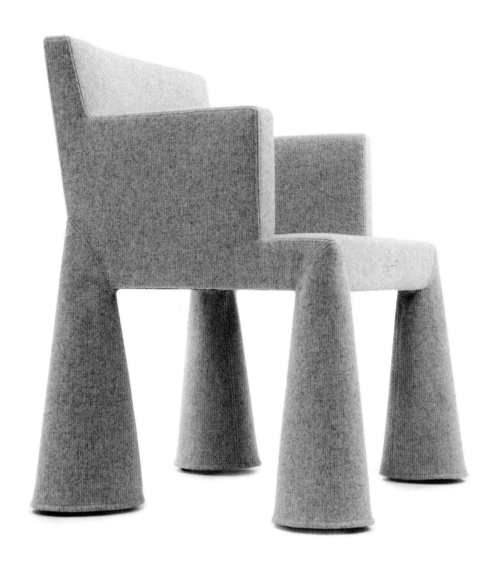

VIP CHAIR, 2000

Metal frame, foam, upholstery

DESIGNER Marcel Wanders, b. 1963

Marcel Wanders Studio, Netherlands

MANUFACTURER Moooi, Netherlands

PHOTOGRAPHY Maarten van Houten

Marcel Wanders's VIP chair reconfigures the lowly slipcover into a high-style garment. In place of the "shabby chic" coverups used to mask worn or unsightly furnishings, VIP wears a close-fitting, precisely tailored suit that never droops or sags. The outer garment appears to stand almost on its own, hovering above the floor.

TINO STOOL, 1999

Aluminum, TechnoGel

DESIGNER   Alessandro Scarpellini Piva

MANUFACTURER   Fontana Arte, Italy

TechnoGel, developed for the health-care industry in the
1970s, typically is used in wheelchairs or hospital beds to
support the body with minimal friction. Designers have
adopted this soft polyurethane material for its cool yet
fleshy translucence. The Tino stool is padded with
TechnoGel; the armrests rise up like protective guardrails.

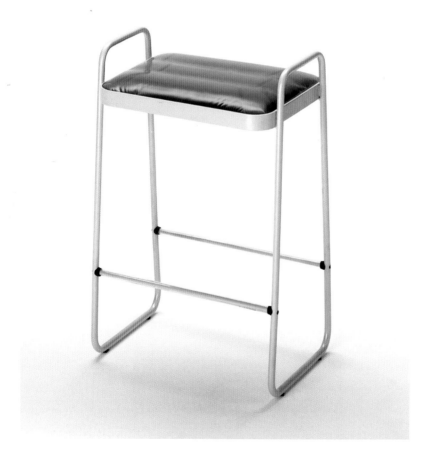

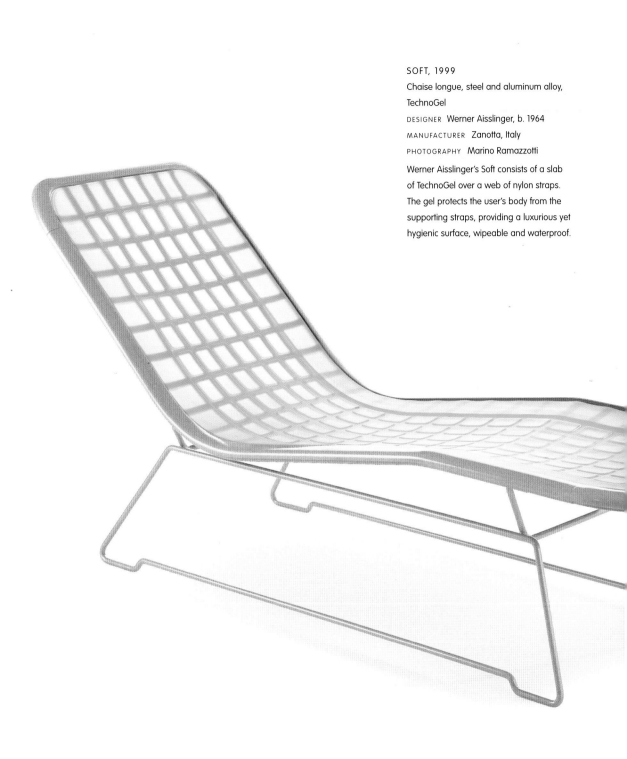

SOFT, 1999

Chaise longue, steel and aluminum alloy, TechnoGel

DESIGNER Werner Aisslinger, b. 1964

MANUFACTURER Zanotta, Italy

PHOTOGRAPHY Marino Ramazzotti

Werner Aisslinger's Soft consists of a slab of TechnoGel over a web of nylon straps. The gel protects the user's body from the supporting straps, providing a luxurious yet hygienic surface, wipeable and waterproof.

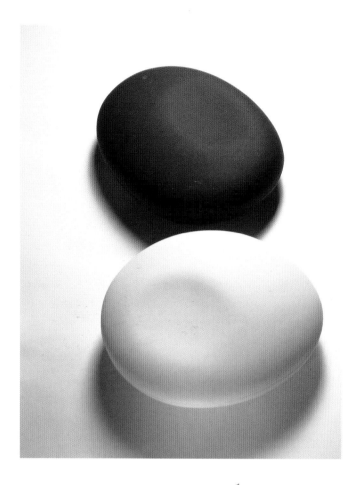

CUSH, 2001
Cushion, self-skinning polyurethane foam

DESIGNERS Pablo Pardo, b. 1962
Tonita Abeyta, b. 1965

MANUFACTURER PABLO, San Francisco

PHOTOGRAPHY Jeffrey Newberry

The Cush pillows by Pablo Pardo and Tonita Abeyta support the body in ways traditional pillows do not, by reflecting the body's curves with subtle indentations. Each polyurethane foam cushion is self-skinning, meaning that the aluminum mold is first sprayed with a coating to match the color of the polyurethane foam. As the foam expands, it bonds with the spray coating to create an integral skin.

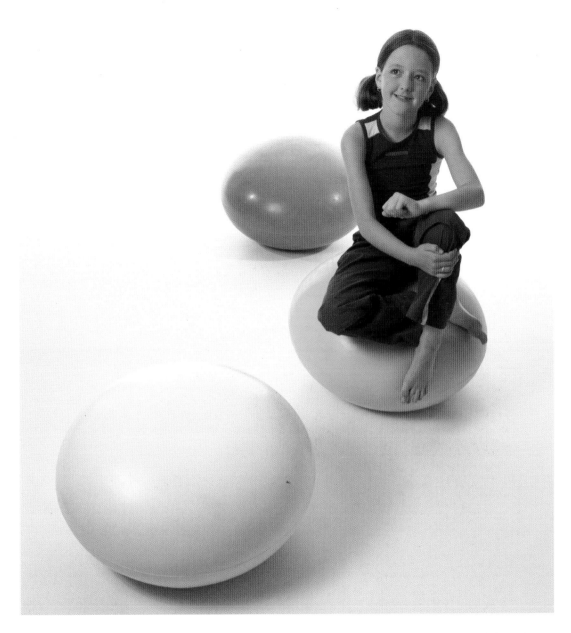

PILL, 2000

Seating, polyethylene foam with rubberlike coating

DESIGNERS Jan Melis, b. 1966
Ben Oostrum, b. 1960

MANUFACTURER M.N.O., Netherlands

PHOTOGRAPHY Hans Oostrum

The Pill chair by Jan Melis and Ben Oostrum is made from soft foam, skinned with a rubbery coat of polyethylene. The Pill serves as informal seating, like a giant pillow, easily moved by children and others. Foam-based furnishings like these are all flesh and no bones, lacking any internal armature of wood or metal. The padding materials become both surface and structure.

AIR ONE, 2000
Seating, polypropylene
DESIGNER   Ross Lovegrove, b. 1958
MANUFACTURER   Edra, Italy
PHOTOGRAPHY   Emilio Tremolada

Ross Lovegrove's Air One is a stackable chair made from the foam material ordinarily used to create packing for computers and other equipment. Lovegrove considered this humble, light material to be as suitable for forming into furniture as other plastics, such as polyurethane. A base material is exploited in its naked state.

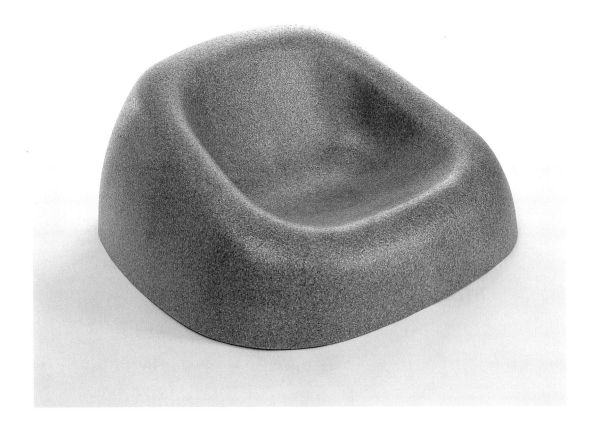

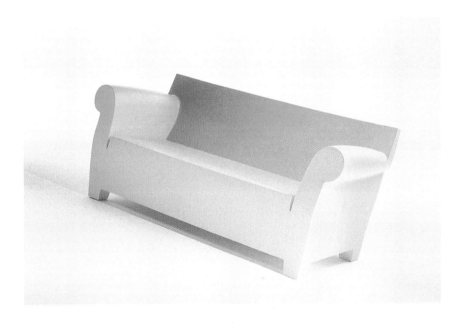

BUBBLE CLUB, 2000

Sofa, polyethylene

DESIGNER Philippe Starck, b. 1949

MANUFACTURER Kartell, Italy

Philippe Starck's Bubble Club sofa is a hollow plastic skin that
mimics the lines of traditional upholstered furniture. The lightweight
Bubble Club sofas and chairs can be used outdoors, where the
mock formality of their profiles is especially endearing. Belying their
scale and apparent mass, these full-sized pieces can be moved
around as casually as ordinary patio furniture.

HI-PAD, 1999

Chair, multidensity polyurethane foam, beech plywood,
fabric, satined steel, rubber

DESIGNER Jasper Morrison, b. 1959

MANUFACTURER Cappellini, Italy

PHOTOGRAPHY Studio Bitetto & Chimenti

The bulging forms of Jasper Morrison's Hi-Pad chair
protrude from the upholstery like anatomical implants.

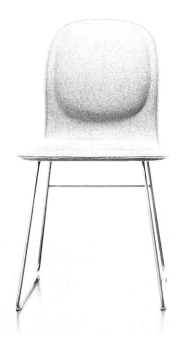
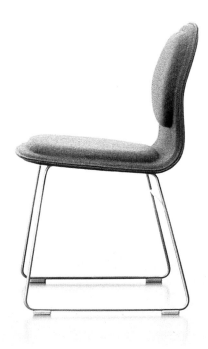

SHELL, 1999
Chair, polyamide, elastin
DESIGNER Riccardo Giovanetti, b. 1967
MANUFACTURER Fontana Arte, Italy

The clefts in Riccardo Giovanetti's Shell chair recall grooves in the flesh of the body. The fabric is bonded to the underlying foam.

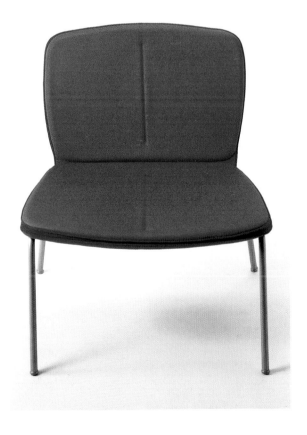

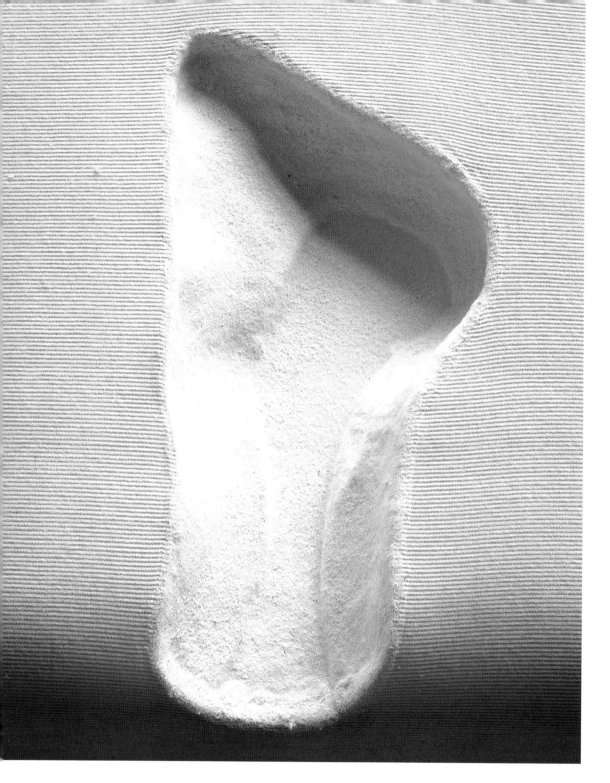

(DETAIL)

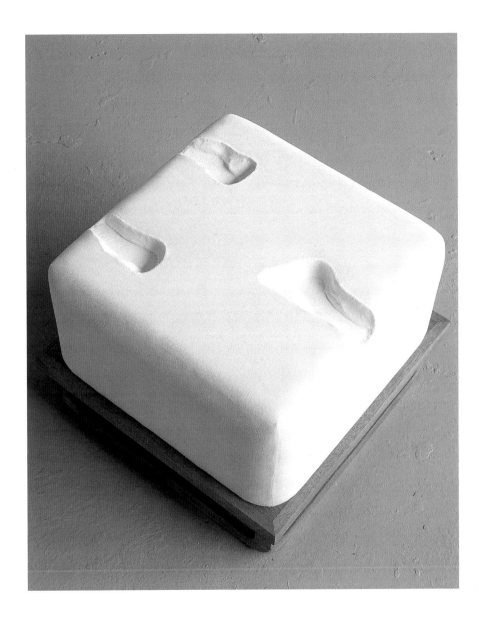

OTTOMAN (CUSTOMIZED
FOR K. FISCHER), 2001

Wood, foam, fabric, rubber, flocking, mahogany

DESIGNER Timothy McLoughlin, b. 1979

Senior thesis project, Maryland Institute
College of Art, Baltimore

PHOTOGRAPHY Dan Meyers

This ottoman is a pristine white cube that has been physically violated. Upholstered in fragile white fabric, the surface of the stool appears gouged with a path of footprints. McLoughlin has inserted rubber castings of footprints into the stool's foam padding, suturing them into place with the care of a surgeon and covering the scars with flocking.

CUBE, 1998

Table, balsa wood, resin, plastic

DESIGNER Elizabeth Paige Smith, b. 1968

MANUFACTURER Elizabeth Paige Smith Design, Los Angeles

PHOTOGRAPHY Lynn Campbell

Elizabeth Paige Smith's Cube table is a block of balsa wood interred in a deep coat of resin. While conventional finishes heighten the visual texture of wood, Smith's milky skin provides a palpable layer of protection, a barrier that diffuses our view of the natural material within.

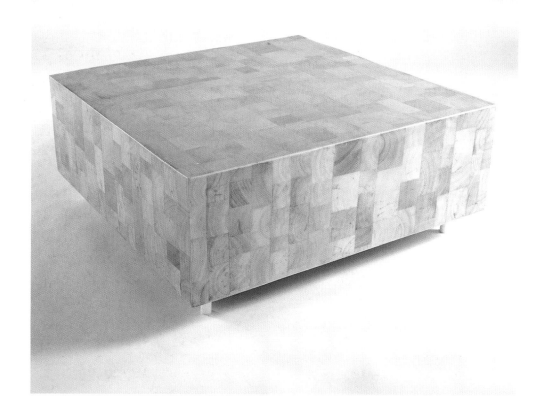

IS, 1999
Table, stained beech, fabric,
soft polyurethane
DESIGNER Marco Ferreri
MANUFACTURER BPA International, Italy
PHOTOGRAPHY Dan Meyers

The top of this table by Marco Ferreri consists of a thin layer of stained beech veneer padded with soft polyurethane. The subtle bulge in the table top subverts our expectations of wood. The exposed edge of the table design draws attention to the skinlike construction of plywood.

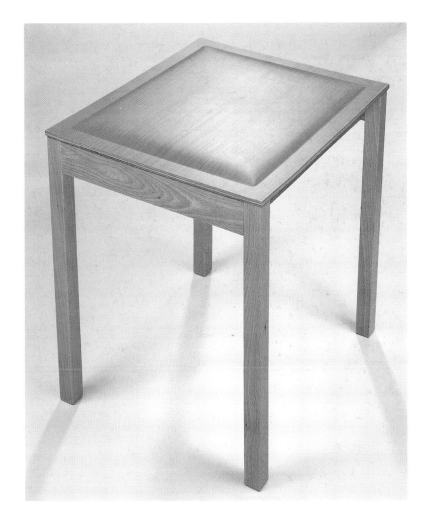

warps
+
folds

SKIN is a two-dimensional surface that wraps around the volumes of the body. Sometimes it is taut, clinging tightly to the musculature beneath, and sometimes it is slack, hanging in loose folds. Fashion often celebrates excess material, finding beauty in wrinkles and creases, as surfaces eddy around the body or take on their own dimensionality.

Paper, a flat, flimsy surface, can be cut and folded into structures that enclose space and carry weight. In architecture and furniture, flat materials are folded or warped to create load-bearing structures, objects that are all surface. Skins weave through space, transforming from inside to outside, top to bottom, ceiling to floor, seat to leg.

LAUGHING EYE, 2000
Photograph

PHOTOGRAPHY   Elinor Carucci, b. 1971
COURTESY OF   Ricco/Maresca Gallery, New York

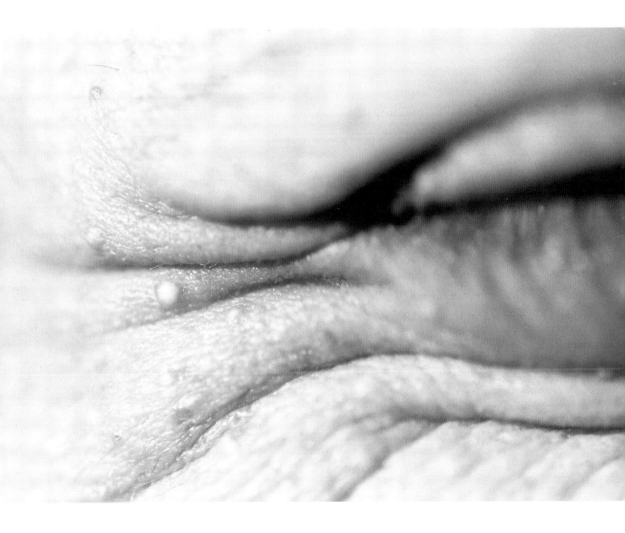

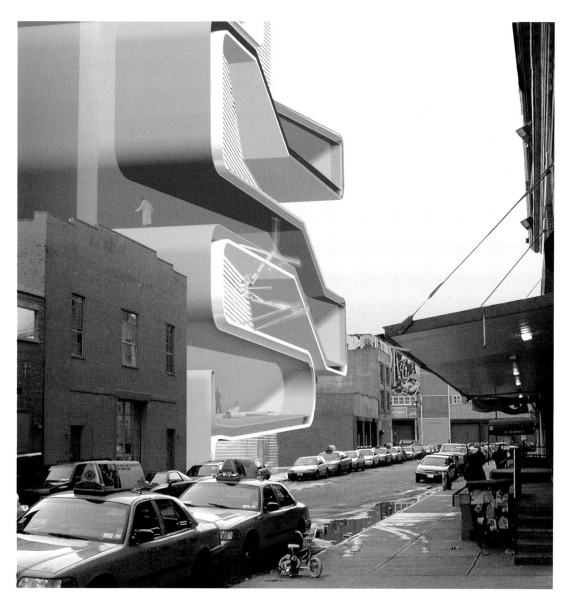

EYEBEAM ATELIER/MUSEUM OF ART
AND TECHNOLOGY COMPETITION,
NEW YORK CITY, 2001
Digital renderings

DESIGNERS Elizabeth Diller, b. 1954
Ricardo Scofidio, b. 1935
Diller + Scofidio, New York

PROJECT LEADER Charles Renfro

TEAM Dirk Hebel, Deane Simpson, Gabriele Heindl,
David Huang, Matthew Johnson, Reto Geisler,
Alex Haw

Diller + Scofidio's competition entry for the Eyebeam Atelier/Museum
of Art and Technology addresses the integration of various programs:
museum, theater, school, and production facility. The design starts
from a simple premise: a pliable ribbon locates production (atelier)
on one side, and presentation (museum/theater) on the other. The
ribbon undulates from side to side as it climbs vertically from the
street. The floor becomes wall, turns into floor, turns into wall, and so
on. With each change of direction, the ribbon enfolds a production
space or presentation space. At various points, the building's
functions infiltrate each other. The ribbon is two-ply, with a technical
space between layers that houses the building's "nervous system."

"The adjacency of a brightly lit atelier space of experimentation and the theatrical ambience of a multimedia installation may raise the question, which one is spectacle? Residents and visitors will observe one another as they move fluidly through the building, sometimes on parallel paths separated by a transparent prophylactic, sometimes crossing paths, sometimes merging paths and sharing programs."
—Diller + Scofidio

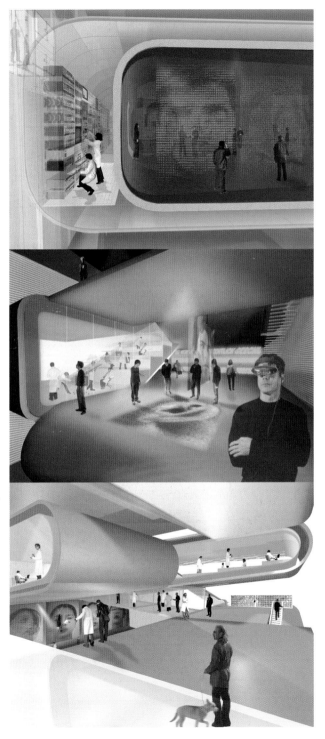

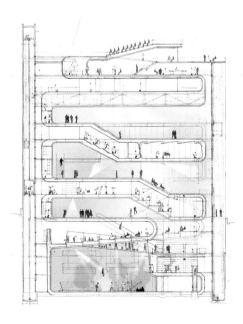

PAPER WALL, 2000

DESIGNERS Stephen Cassell, b. 1963

Adam Yarinsky, b. 1962

ARO (Architecture Research Office), New York

TEAM Scott Abrahams, Matt Azen, Alan Bruton

LASER CUTTER V Class Universal Laser Systems

Support for this project was provided by the New York

State Council on the Arts and Artists Space Gallery

PHOTOGRAPHY Reid Freeman

In this experimental project, the architectural firm ARO used a computer-driven laser cutter to create a dimensional wall structure entirely out of paper. The laser cuts and scores in ways that cannot be achieved by hand, transforming paper's material qualities. The Paper Wall was exhibited at Artists Space in February 2000.

"Designers can now work directly with computer programs to produce nearly finished products. The technology is changing the creative thought process of design, paradoxically bringing it closer to its craft roots."
—Adam Yarinsky and Stephen Cassell, ARO

COLORADO HOUSE,
TELLURIDE, COLORADO, 1999

Detail of custom weathering Cor-ten steel shingles

DESIGNERS Stephen Cassell

Adam Yarinsky

ARO (Architecture Research Office), New York

PROJECT ARCHITECT John Quale

TEAM Scott Abrahams, Matt Azen, Tom Jenkinson, Monica Rivera, Martha Skinner, Kim Yao, Innes Yates

PHOTOGRAPHY Paul Warchol

The exterior walls of a vacation house in Colorado, designed by ARO, are covered with custom-cut shingles of Cor-ten steel. Changes in the overlapping pattern of the shingles give a dynamic quality to the surface of the walls, with the north-facing walls having a more pronounced diagonal pattern than the south-facing walls. The shingles comprise the outer layer of a rain-screen wall system.

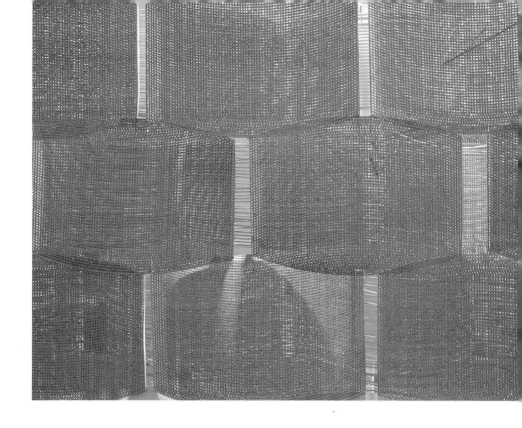

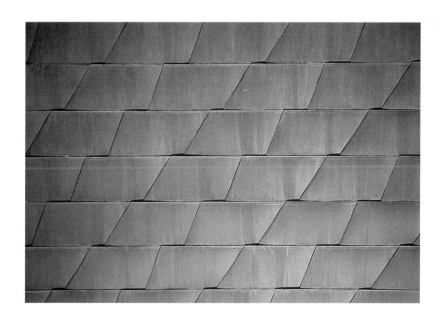

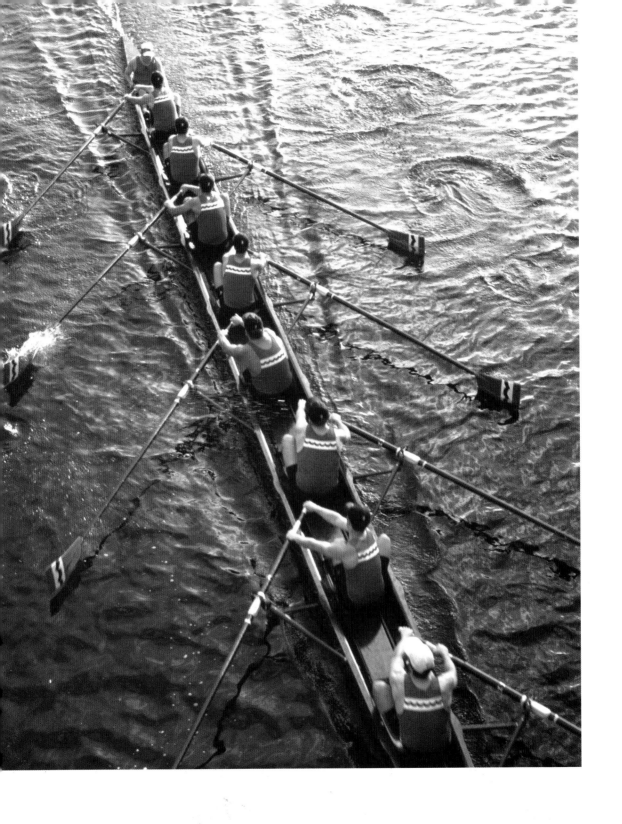

RESOLUTE: THE 8, 2001

Eight-seat rowing shell, carbon fiber,
Nomex honeycomb (Kevlar paper dipped in
phenolic resin)

DESIGNER Jim Taylor, Dirk Kramers, Eric Goetz
and Steve Gladstone

MANUFACTURER Resolute Racing Shells,
Bristol, Rhode Island

PHOTOGRAPHY Billy Black

A composite of light, strong materials are used to
construct this 60-foot-long racing shell, which
weighs less than 250 pounds. The strength of the
vessel derives from the curvature of the thin skin
as well as from the materials used.

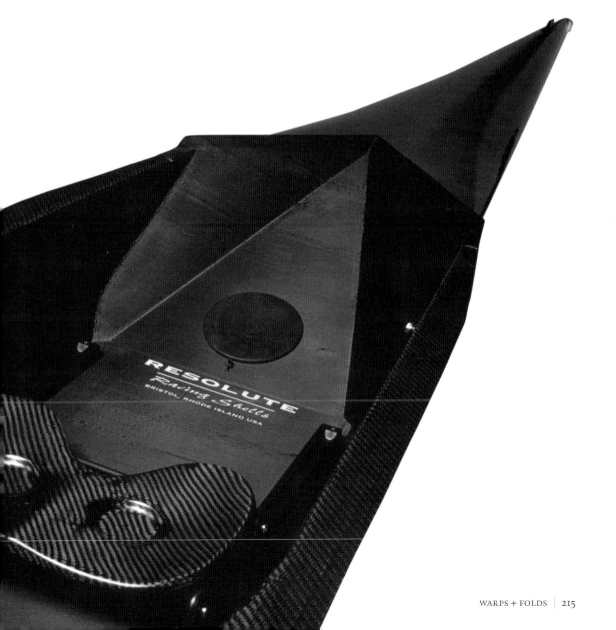

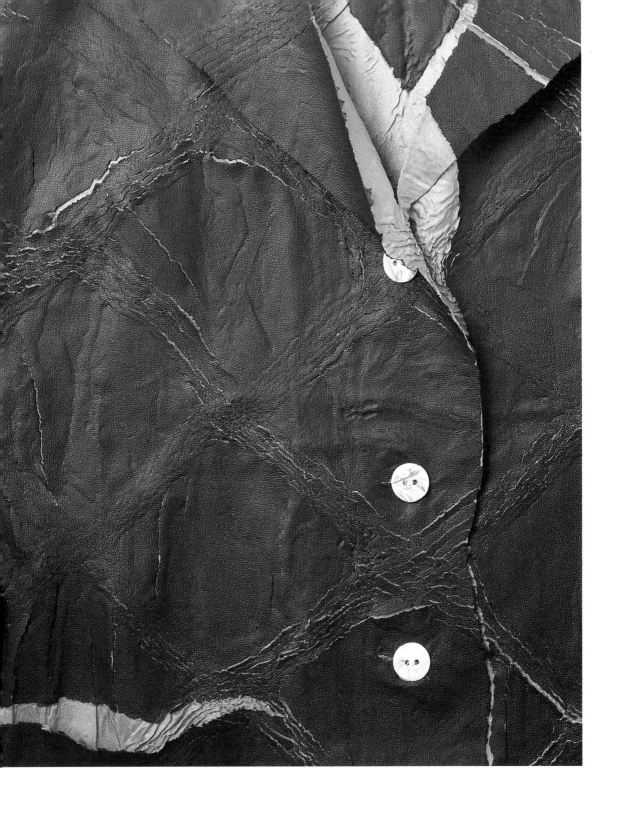

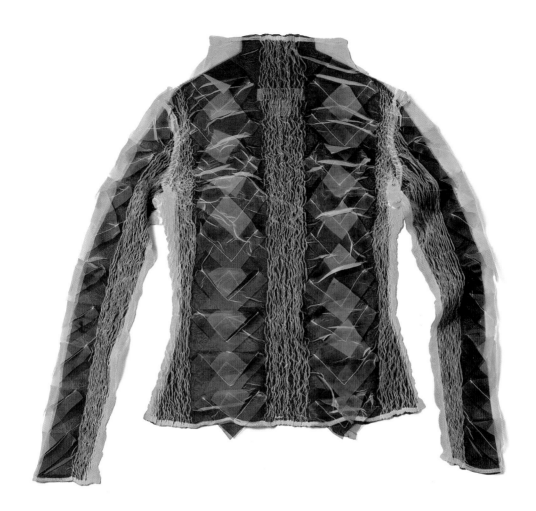

YOSHIKI HISHINUMA,
FALL COLLECTION, 2001

Garments, nylon, vinyl

DESIGNER   Yoshiki Hishinuma, b. 1958
MANUFACTURER Hishinuma Association, Japan
PHOTOGRAPHY Matt Flynn

Yoshiki Hishinuma's clothes use a traditional Japanese technique in which a thin fabric is knotted or sewn, sometimes in multiple layers. The fabric is then shrunk, causing it to pucker. In some of Hishinuma's pieces, a sheet of vinyl is laminated to the translucent layers beneath; the vinyl is allowed to crack, exposing the delicate flesh below the broken skin. These pieces explore the beauty and complexity of wrinkles, tears, and imperfections.

IMAGES CONTINUE ON FOLLOWING PAGES

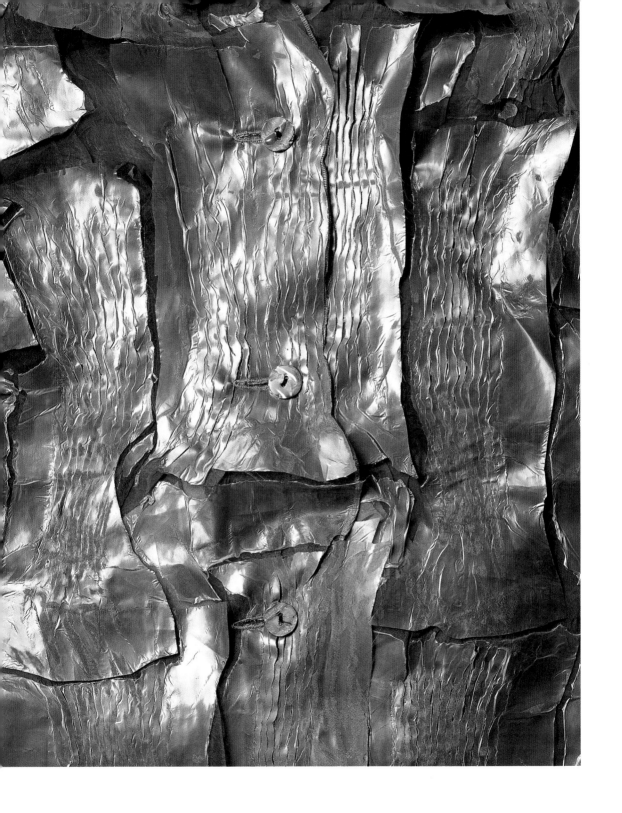

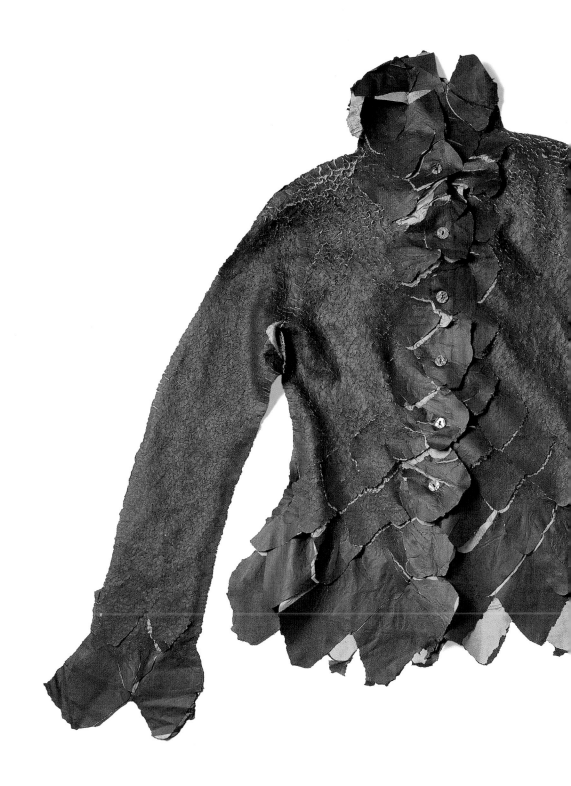

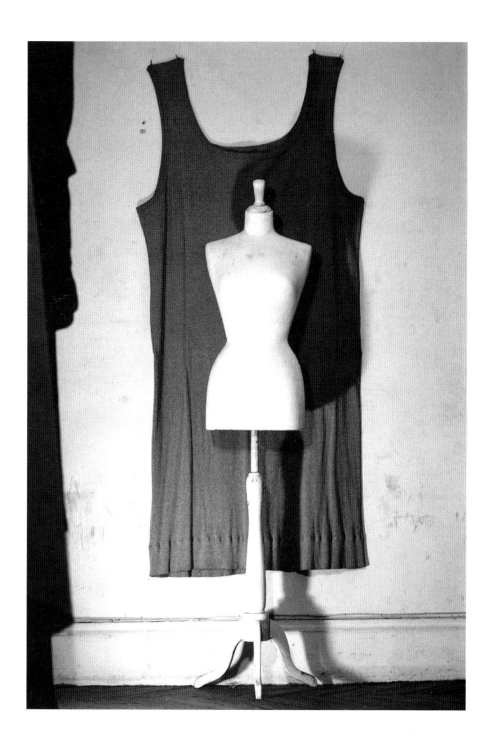

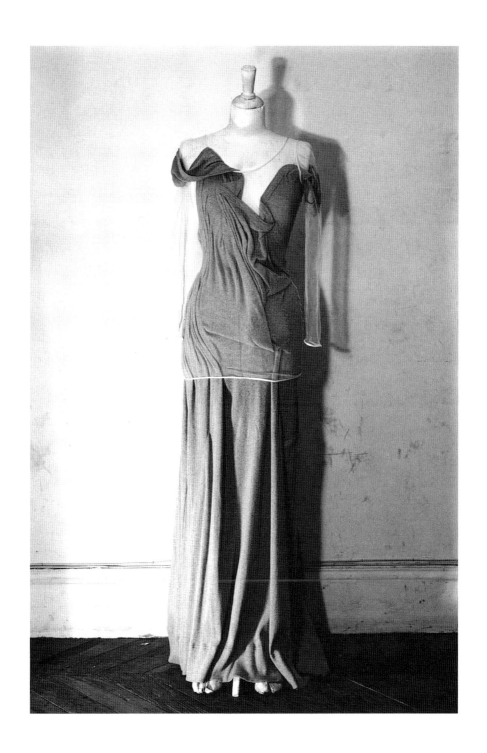

PREVIOUS PAGES

XXXL VEST WITH T-SHIRT, 1991

Cotton, nylon

DESIGNER Martin Margiela

Maison Martin Margiela, Paris

PHOTOGRAPHY Tatsuya Kitayama, Paris

Belgian designer Martin Margiela was a leader of the "deconstructionist" movement that reshaped the international fashion world in the 1980s and 1990s. Margiela is known for taking the generic elements of fashion and reconfiguring their scale, function, and physical structure. Here, an enormous t-shirt—larger than any human being—is worn beneath a fine net sheath. As the excess skin of the t-shirt swirls around the body, a nascent classicism emerges out of base, industrial materials.

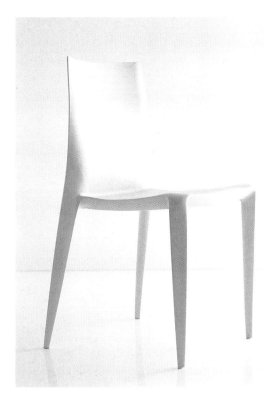

BELLINI CHAIR, 1998

Injection-molded plastic

DESIGNER Mario Bellini, b. 1935

MANUFACTURER Heller, United States

PHOTOGRAPHY Pietro Carrieri

The supple, erotic Bellini Chair is made from a single skin of continuously curving plastic.

ISSEY MIYAKE BOW AND
TUMMY HOLIDAY BAGS, 1997
Packaging, extruded Cleartint™
polypropylene
DESIGNER Karim Rashid, b. 1960
MANUFACTURER Issey Miyake, Japan

Karim Rashid's packaging for Issey Miyake is made from thin translucent plastic. The design exploits the flexibilty of the material, as gentle curves replace the conventional rectilinear box. Designed for use in Issey Miyake stores, the folded packages nest against each other like cells, membrane to membrane. A single pattern can create either form, depending on how it is folded.

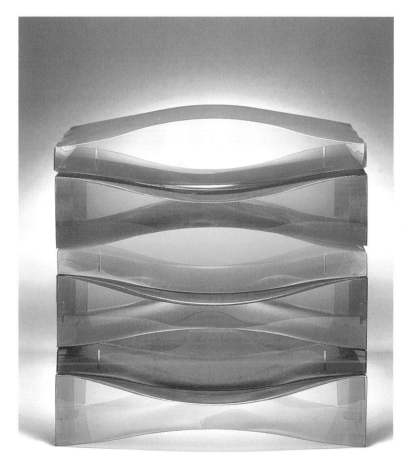

FOLDER, 2000

Chairs, polypropylene

DESIGNER Stefan Schöning, b. 1968

Stefan Schöning Industrial Design, Antwerp

MANUFACTURER Polyline, Belgium

PHOTOGRAPHY Sigfrid Eggers

The Folder chair is made from polypropylene, a paperlike, flexible plastic. The chair is folded together like a work of origami and shipped assembled. The thin planes curve gently, softening the angularity of the folded material.

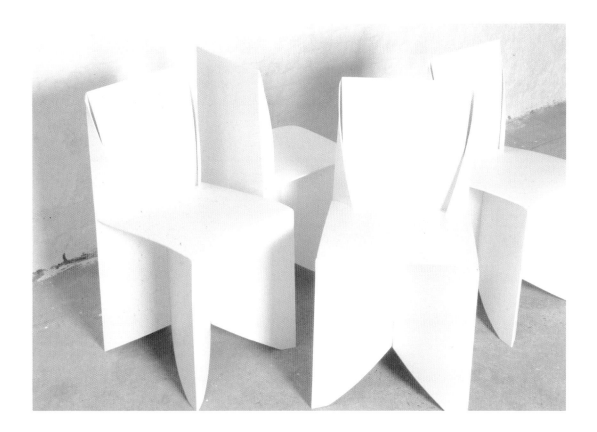

VOXIA: ECO, 1999
Chair, laminated (form pressed) beech wood
DESIGNER   Peter Karpf, b. 1940
MANUFACTURER   Iform, Sweden
PHOTOGRAPHY   Johan Kalén

The Voxia line of chairs, designed by Peter Karpf, is made from planes of laminated beech wood that are cut and bent into structural forms. The back, seat, and legs are produced and combined in one continuous process. The material, peeled veneer, is made by rotary-cutting the whole tree trunk—the tree is, in principle, unrolled into a sheet of skin, from outside in, a process that yields minimum waste.

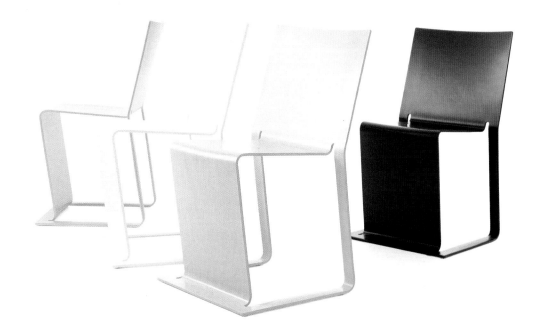

MITRE FOLD STOOL, 2001

Prototype, rubber, plywood

DESIGNERS   Charles Lazor, b. 1964

John Christakos, b. 1964

Maurice Blanks, b. 1964

MANUFACTURER   Blu Dot, Minneapolis

PHOTOGRAPHY   Ryanne Williams

This folding stool is made from a sheet of plywood laminated with rubber. The plywood is precisely mitred with a CNC (computer numeric control) tool, which makes cuts specified directly from the designer's CAD (computer aided design) drawings. The stool is manufactured, packaged, and shipped flat. After the stool is folded into place by the consumer, the self-skinning foam seat is set into place.

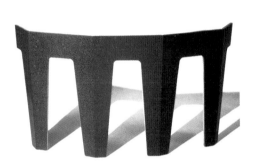
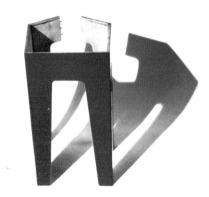
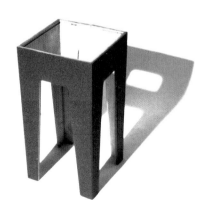
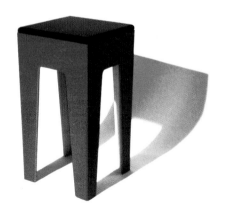

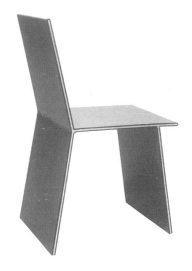

TRUDY, 2001
Chair, aluminum frame covered with
polyurethane foam
DESIGNER Michael Solis, b. 1969
MANUFACTURER Dune, New York

This chair by Michael Solis is made from thin
planes of aluminum sandwiched between
resilient layers of foam. The conjunction of
diverse materials is revealed along the edges of
the piece, where soft and rigid skins meet.

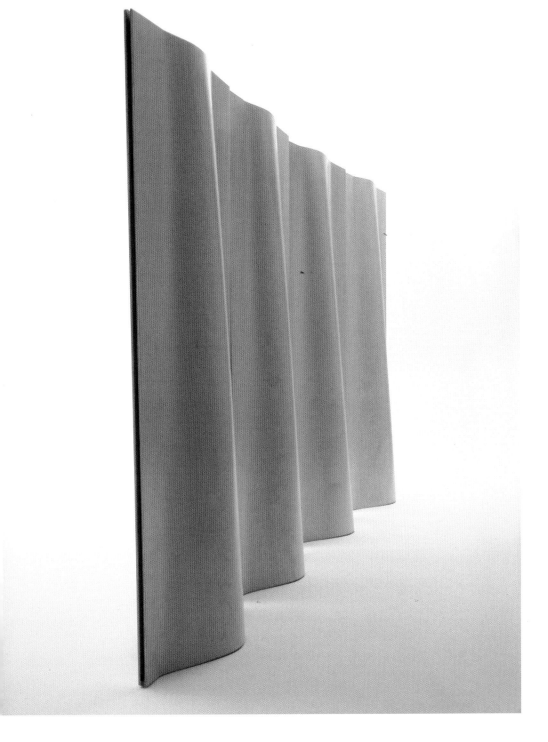

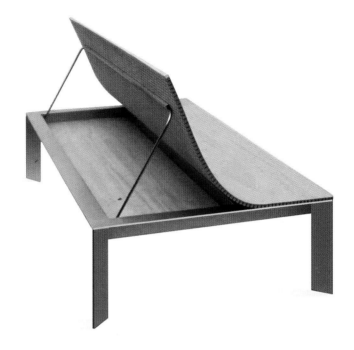

UP, 2001 LEFT

Screen, Coverflex plywood

DESIGNER Paolo Ulian, b. 1961

MANUFACTURER

BBB Bonacina, Italy

PHOTOGRAPHY

Massimo Colombo

Paolo Ulian's UP screen is made from flexible plywood. The screen is packed flat. To make it a freestanding screen, the user simply compresses it on its vertical sides until an inner mechanism locks it open.

CABRIOLET, 2001 RIGHT

Furniture, aluminum frame with Coverflex plywood top covered in Tanganyika walnut

DESIGNER Paolo Ulian

MANUFACTURER

Fontana Arte, Milan

PHOTOGRAPHY

Amendolaggine e Barracchia

Paolo Ulian's Cabriolet is topped with a flexible sheet of wood. In its closed, horizontal position, the piece is a table. The surface peels upward, however, to become the seat and back of a bench. A material that appears to be rigid and fixed proves to be flexible, enabling the object to transform its function.

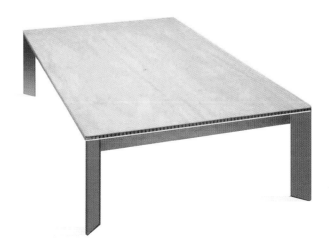

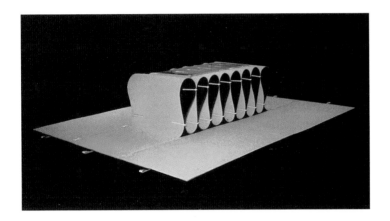

FRAISE, 2000
Furniture prototype, soft foam
DESIGNER Ilan Korren, b. 1964
Appel Permanent V.I.A., Paris, 1999
Prototype made in Israel
PHOTOGRAPHY Samuel Gomez

Ilan Korren's Fraise is made from sheets of foam
folded into loops. The object, whose name refers
to a traditional ruffled collar, serves as a rug, table,
and magazine rack.

FELT STOOL NO. 7, 2000
Prototype, polyester felt, nylon, aluminum
DESIGNERS Robert Moorhead, b. 1972
Granger Moorhead, b. 1969
Moorhead & Moorhead, New York
Andy Kurrasch, Senior Project Engineer,
Herman Miller Red
PHOTOGRAPHY Robert Moorhead

Architects and industrial designers Robert and Granger Moorhead created this simple stool by folding a single sheet of heavy industrial felt and pinning it together at just three points. The deep folds are erotic and mysterious. Like a fortune cookie or an alien cocoon, the stool appears to harbor an intriguing secret. The stool is being developed in 100 percent felt for the Herman Miller Red line of office furnishings.

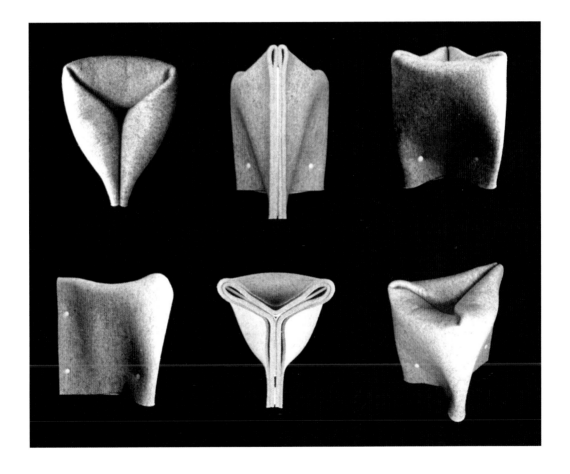

glossary of materials

THE MODERN OBJECT world is constructed from a vast inventory of materials, some harvested from the field or forest, others derived from the skin and hair of animals. The materials most identified with twentieth- and twenty-first-century design, however, are synthesized from petroleum, silicon, and chemicals, creating that amorphous family of substances known, generally, as "plastics." In 1979 world-wide production of plastic outstripped production of steel, a watershed in the ascendent economy of synthetics. Catalogued here are a few of the materials used by designers today. They provide the artificial surfaces, simulated skins, and foam-based flesh of contemporary objects.

The glossary is written by Grace Jeffers.
Contributions by Randi Mates are marked
with her initials.

GRACE JEFFERS
with contributions by Randi Mates

Aerogel, sometimes called "blue smoke," is a silicon-based solid with a porous, spongelike structure invented in 1930. In the United States, Aerogel is produced by the Jet Propulsion Laboratory, in California. Because 99 percent of its volume is empty space, it is one thousand times less dense than glass (another silicon-based solid). With a weight only three times that of air, Aerogel is extraordinarily light as well as strong and transparent. NASA's Stardust space mission (1999) used Aerogel to capture comet dust. In 1999 Aerogel insulated the Mars Rover. Here on earth, Aerogel's insulating capability can be translated into a number of consumer products—oven doors, refrigerators, picnic coolers, and even clothing. Airglass, in Sweden, is currently producing windows using Aerogel, which could significantly increase energy efficiency. One pane has the equivalent thermal insulating quality of ten to twenty glass panes, and a 1-inch thickness can protect a human hand from a blow torch. In the future, Aerogel could reduce the size of the computer chip by providing a smaller, more compact substitute for traditional silicon.

Decorative high-pressure laminate (HPL) is composed of stacked layers of kraft paper that have been impregnated with plastic resin (the same resin as in Bakelite) and fused into a solid homogenous product with pressure and heat. The surface, or decorative layer, is a printed sheet of white paper or a solid sheet of colored paper coated with melamine. The material commonly is referred to as "plastic laminate," a name that is somewhat misleading, as 87 percent of the material is actually paper.

Early uses of plastic laminate—as components for radio interiors and as coverings for electrical wires—were purely industrial. Decorative uses were not explored until the 1920s. The first plastic laminate, Micarta, was developed at Westinghouse in Pittsburgh in 1908. Shortly thereafter, two disgruntled Westinghouse employees, Herbert A. Faber and Daniel J. O'Connor, left to form their own renegade laminate company, and in 1913 they formed the Formica Insulation Company. In 1927 Formica was awarded a patent for a decorative laminate, topped with a colorful layer. In the 1930s the material was the preferred surface for elegant bars and nightclubs, because it was impervious to both alcohol and cigarette burns. The material was expensive and available only to the building trade until the mid-1940s, when Formica set out to make its name synonymous with the material, much to the chagrin of the seventeen other U.S. laminate manufacturers. Today, just five U.S. manufacturers produce more than three billion square feet of laminate for domestic consumption. Laminates are commonly used on kitchen countertops or as a finishing surface on furniture. Historic uses include everything from airplane propellers to snow and water skis. Laminates with a protective coating containing aluminum oxides are currently used as flooring.

Electroluminescent film was discovered in the 1930s, when electroluminescent (EL) technology was most commonly used in exit signage. Since then, it has been used to backlight wristwatches and pagers. EL films consist of three thin layers of plastic: a middle layer with a phosphorous powder coating, and two outer conductive layers, one of which is transparent. As an electric current passes from one conductive layer to another, the phosphorous powder glows and emits light. EL films are now so thin that display signs can be set flush against a wall, unlike conventional backlit signs. They can be wrapped around corners and complex architectural shapes or suspended from ceilings. In addition to being thin and flexible, EL film lighting uses very little power.

Fake fur has been made for centuries, and was originally fabricated out of high piles of cut natural fibers, such as silk. The first synthetic pile fabric, Dynel, was composed of modacrylic fibers and was manufactured by the Union Carbide Company in 1949. Though Dynel is no longer in production, the composition of fake fur has remained consistent. A modacrylic fiber is any synthetic fiber that, by weight, contains between 35 and 85 percent of the chemical compound acrylonitrile. Synthetic furs are mothproof, water repellent, and resistant to chemical damage.

Early fake furs primarily provided cheap alternatives to real furs. By the late 1960s, environmental activism instigated a public movement against the wearing of real furs. Fun furs, dyed in a spectrum of unusual colors and cut in trendy styles, became popular in the 1970s. People for the Ethical Treatment of Animals (PETA), founded in 1980, staged extensive public awareness campaigns agitating against the use of real fur, creating a fake fur boom in the middle of the decade. Fake fur's recent popularity has more to do with the pile's verisimilitude than the flagrant display of fakeness prized in the 1970s. In the late 1990s, fake fur was often featured in home furnishings magazines as a luxurious surface that softened the harsh edges of modernistic interiors. A throwaway luxury as well as an economical substitute, fake furs continue to go in and out of fashion. R M

Latex is a milky secretion from the rubber tree (Hevea brasiliensis), originally found in Brazil. Ducts containing latex run just below the surface of the tree bark. If a thin layer of bark is shaved, latex flows from the ducts and can be collected in a container. Left alone, the collected material will become a lump of rubber, but if it is mixed

with an anticoagulant such as ammonia, it becomes flexible. Ten percent of all natural rubber produced is made into latex, which is used in balloons, baby bottle nipples, rubber bands, medical gloves, and condoms. Since the late 1940s, it has been used in paint because it provides flexibility, durability, adhesion, color retention, and resistance to chemicals. Synthetic or artificial latex is made by dispersing reclaimed synthetic rubber, natural rubber, or rubberlike plastics in water. Artificial latex is commonly used as a component of adhesives.

Lenticular printing was invented in the late 1930s by a company called VariVue, which coined the terms "lenticular" and "winkies" to refer to their products. VariVue produced stereographic and animated lenticular images for everything from Cracker Jack prizes and billboard advertisements to postcards and political buttons. A lenticular image is a thin plastic sheet composed of a series of parallel lenses on top of an interlaced image. The lenses allow the viewer to see different sections of the underlying image at different viewing angles. The interlaced image can be either different angles of the same subject or a completely different image. The lenticular plastic filters the view so that only one image is visible at a time, but as the viewer's head moves from side to side, the succession of images appears to be either moving or changing from one image to another. Lenticular images are used for a variety of products, from toys, wallpaper, and textiles to conversion tools (Celsius to Fahrenheit, feet to miles, and so on). In the 1980s the Secret Service conducted a study that showed that lenticular images are the most difficult to reproduce— more difficult than holograms—and began using them for security badges and ID cards.

Naugahyde, developed by U.S. Rubber in 1917, was the first rubber-based imitation leather. The name of the material derives from its place of origin (Naugatuck, Connecticut) and its resemblance to animal hide. The earliest uses of Naugahyde included upholstery for railroad cars and automobiles, footwear, luggage, and handbags. Initially, Naugahyde was a mixture of ground leather and rubber pressed onto a flexible, synthetic film that was treated with an adhesive. The entire composition was then waterproofed and, depending on its end-use, embossed to look like leather. Before World War II, however, rumored rubber shortages prompted U.S. Rubber to develop a formula that replaced Naugahyde's rubber with vinyl. The resulting durable product was used extensively by the American military during the war for both apparel and transport cover. Postwar advances included an expanded range of colors and finishes, as well as "breathable" versions that were considered more hygienic and comfortable on the skin. The most significant postwar advance, however, was the introduction of increasingly elastic backings, which allowed the material to easily sheathe a wider variety of forms.

In 1967, the new patent-holders of Naugahyde, UniRoyal Corporation, launched a marketing campaign that told the "history" of a fictitious Nauga beast. This lummoxlike creature reputedly dated back to the ancient world and had a "self-shedding" hide, which made Naugahyde a "cruelty-free" fabric. While many people knew that the Nauga was an ad executive's creation, the myth of a Nauga beast persists in contemporary folklore.

Naugahyde uses have evolved to suit modern consumer needs. The wheelchair industry has created Naugahyde slipcovers that do not irritate the sitter's skin. The sound-absorbent fabric is also used in recording studios. Its water-resistance makes Naugahyde a favorite for both interior and exterior uses on boats. Because it is an inexpensive and low-maintenance alternative to leather, it is also widely used as upholstery in homes and for public seating. New versions of Naugahyde are so resistant to fire that only the surface layer is damaged by flames, serving to wholly protect the material beneath. R M

Nylon, synthesized from petrochemicals, is a superpolymer that can be spun into long, flexible fibers. Developed in 1934 by DuPont chemist Wallace D. Caruthers, nylon was the first wholly synthetic fiber ever manufactured. Nylon made its official public debut in a variety of products at the San Francisco Golden Gate International Exhibition in 1939. Erotic, lustrous, form-fitting, and sheer, nylon stockings grabbed the public's

attention and were an immediate success. Shortly thereafter, the U.S. government triggered national hysteria when it requisitioned all nylon production for the World War II effort.

Nylon's popularity remained strong during the latter half of the century, despite the introduction of numerous other synthetic fibers. No longer an object of frenzied desire, it became so common as to be almost invisible. Found in toothbrushes, clothing, gas tank liners, plastic packaging, computer hardware, and dollar bills, nylon has become a modern original, its man-made origins unimportant in the face of its overarching utility. R M

Pleather, or plastic leather, is a synthetic fabric made from polyurethane or PVC that resembles leather. Often used in clothing, it is less expensive, lighter weight, and more versatile than leather because it can be easily embossed, embroidered, and dyed. Today pleather is softer, thinner, and more supple than its earliest versions in the 1970s, but because it does not breathe well, it can be hot to wear. Some manufacturers combine it with cotton or viscose for increased ventilation.

Polyethylene, the first inexpensive plastic, began production in the 1930s, but didn't gain wide acceptance until Earl Tupper, in the first years after World War II, molded it into his famous storage containers. Tupper praised the material because it withstood kitchen stresses such as knife cuts and near-boiling temperatures. In 1958, American manufacturers converted 920 million pounds of polyethylene into countless consumer items, from squeeze to inexpensive laundry baskets. By 1960, packaging alone consumed 300,000 tons. Today, polyethylene remains one of the most common plastics.

Polyethylenes are waxy, translucent thermoplastic polymers that are lightweight, chemical resistant, tough, and relatively inexpensive—properties that make this plastic ideal for containers for such common items as laundry detergent and motor oil. Low Density Polyethylene (LDPE), one of the first polyethylenes to be developed, is a film and is used for grocery bags, dry cleaning bags, and resealable coffee can lids. High Density Polyethylene (HDPE) is more rigid and has more tensile and compressive strength. Pink lawn flamingoes are made from HDPE. Because HDPE is FDA-approved for direct food contact, it is also used for cutting boards.

Polyethylene terephthalate (PET)—the magic material that made plastic soda and water bottles possible—was pioneered as a joint effort between Pepsi and DuPont in 1973. Other permutations include polyethylene rubber, polyethylene wax, and ultra-high-molecular weight polyethylenes, which are more ballistic-repellent than steel.

Polypropylene was invented in Italy by Giulio Natta in the 1950s and became available in the United States in 1957. It is an economical thermoplastic made by a process similar to that used to create polyethylene. But while polyethylene is soft, polypropylene is more rigid. Polypropylene can be used as both a plastic and a fiber. It has good electrical and chemical resistance, which also means stain resistance. As a plastic, it is used in café chairs, milk crates, toolboxes, toilet seats, and prosthetic devices. Because of its high melting point, polypropylene is used for dishwasher-safe food containers and hospital implements that require repeated sterilization. As a fiber, it is used to make indoor-outdoor carpeting because it does not absorb water.

Polyurethane is a group of polyester-based resins that can be made into foams of varying flexibility, from flexible to semiflexible, semirigid, and rigid. Soft polyurethane offers a unique combination of high elasticity and the durability of metal; it is the flexible foam most often used in furniture as seat cushions or mattresses. Lycra, the fiber used in stretch clothing, is also a polyurethane. Because it is highly resistant to abrasion, polyurethane can be used as a durable coating—both decorative and protective.

In 1968 Douglas Deeds created the first "completely abstract, totally synthetic environment in the history of construction" by spraying polyurethane foam into an amorphously shaped room complete with voids for windows and out-croppings for seating. This room was first shown in an exhibition entitled *Plastic for Plastic* at the Museum for Contemporary Crafts in New York. At the same time, Felix Drury experimented with the material to mold cocoonlike habitation pods. The U.S. Bicentennial of 1976 and the restoration of Williamsburg ignited a fashion for historic revivalism in the 1970s. Both the furniture and the architectural molding industries mass-produced decorative carvings such as rosettes, medallions, and ornate faux wood furnishings out of the polyurethane foam. In the 1970s the material became less popular when it was discovered that when it burned, it produced a dense black smoke that was often lethal.

Polyvinyl Chloride, or **PVC**, is a thermoplastic that can be made either flexible or rigid and is chemically nonreactive. It has a wide range of applications and comes in many forms, from foams to sheets, films, and rods. PVC is used in plumbing pipes, lab equipment, and machine parts. It was invented in 1926 by Waldo Semon, a researcher at B. F. Goodrich. At the time, ethylene was considered a useless byproduct of petroleum processing and was usually thrown away. In his experiments, Semon found that he could create a gelatinous substance with a variable elasticity. He also found that the material was highly moldable, waterproof, and fire resistant. While watching his wife make curtains, he realized it could be used like fabric. The company marketed the product under the name Koroseal, and it gained popularity through its use in shower curtains, umbrellas, and raincoats. Today, PVC is second only to polyethylene as the world's most widely used plastic.

Pudgee was developed during the oil crisis of the 1970s. This high-density foam was created by American Charles Yost, using polyurethane techniques and a combination of plant materials and chemicals. Pudgee is used most often as a "smart" seat cushion in the medical, aeronautic, and space industries. With properties of both a foam and a gel, Pudgee has some give as well as a memory; it responds to weight by receiving the impression of the body placed upon it. Therefore, the pressure from seams in the sitter's clothing is transferred to the material's surface rather than pressed into the wearer's skin. Pudgee is often cooler than room temperature and absorbs body moisture, keeping human skin cool and dry. Soft and pliant, Pudgee also eases the sitter's circulation, allowing more comfortable sitting for long periods of time. A hybrid of organic and synthetic materials, Pudgee is more durable and resilient than its individual components and is able to maintain its unique properties in most temperature conditions.

Rubber is available in both organic and inorganic forms. Natural rubber, which is simply the sap from the Hevea tree, was brought to the Western Hemisphere in the early eighteenth century, after an English scientist traveling in the West Indies saw natives playing with bouncing balls. By the mid-nineteenth century, vulcanization, a process through which rubber is heated and made impenetrable, was perfected and patented. Supple, elastic, and pliant, organic rubber was used to make false teeth, tabletops, waterproof high heels, tires, rubber sheeting, and other goods. The utilitarian Macintosh, a waterproof coat made of rubber and cloth, was introduced in 1823. In the twentieth century, the rubber industry sought to make its product fashionable. As early as the 1930s, DuPont began embossing their rubberized fabrics with patterns, in order to both naturalize and modernize the material for the buying public. In the first half of the twentieth century, rubber was thought of as hygienic, durable, practical, and stylish.

Synthetic rubber, or Neoprene, made from acetylene gas waste, was introduced by DuPont in 1931. Advanced development of inorganic rubber did not begin until the start of World War II, when the threat of an inadequate supply forced the chemical industry to seek alternatives. By early 1942, a consortium of rubber producers had created a recipe for synthetic rubber, named GR-S, a blend of butadiene and methyl methacrylate. Synthetic rubber, which soon came to dominate the market, had all of the properties of natural rubber but with increased durability.

Rubber is a malleable, load-bearing, self-healing material that can be used as a laminate with other materials, or on its own. It can be injection-molded in a variety of forms as well as fashioned into sheets. Rubber is now used as cable insulation, bullets, pillows, casing for plumbing equipment, toys, and flooring. Introduced into couture with vinyl in the 1960s, rubber remains popular in fetish wear. Standing in stark contrast to the flesh of the wearer while simultaneously molding to the body, the material becomes an artificial skin, both denying and heightening the corporeality of the body beneath. Still available in both organic and inorganic forms, which are sometimes indistinguishable, rubber eschews popular perceptions of a great divide between the qualities found in synthetic and natural materials.
R M

Silicon is a nonmetallic chemical element—indeed, the second most abundant element in the earth's crust. It has extreme temperature resistance and will maintain its chemical integrity in temperatures ranging from −180°F to 600°F (−118°C to 315°C). Its conductive electric properties make it ideal for switches and keypads in high-tech products like computers or cell phones. Because of its high heat resistance, silicon can also be used in lighting products. Silicone rubber is inert, odorless, tasteless, and stainless, making it ideal for medical and food preparations. It is used in breast implants, freezer ice trays, and flexible baking molds.

TechnoGel, originally produced in the 1970s by Bayer for the medical industry under the name Levagel, is now made by the German company TechnoGel. This polyurethane gel was developed for wound dressings because of its soft, water-adhesive properties. By altering the ratio of ingredients, engineers changed its consistency, creating a rubberlike nonadhesive material for use in wheelchair cushions, pressure-relieving pads, and bicycle seats. Its memory capability allows it to return to its original shape after prolonged exposure to high pressure. Many designers, attracted to TechnoGel's translucency as well as its texture and performance, are experimenting with the material in furniture.

Vinyl is a generic name encompassing a range of materials. The origins of vinyl production are debated. Some reports posit German chemist H. A. Klatt as the first to polymerize the material in 1913. Polyvinyl chloride, or PVC, is a specific type of vinyl, whose invention is widely attributed to a technician at B. F. Goodrich in 1926. A three-step chemical reaction between ethylene and chlorine produces vinyl polymer, a white, dustlike resin that is then combined with other additives to produce specific end products. Because of the natural abundance of chlorine, vinyl is inexpensive—unlike plastics made with petro-chemicals. Vinyl is also versatile, moisture-resistant, long lasting, durable, inherently fire-resistant, and can be made in any color. It can be produced in a flexible form, as in upholstery, as well as in a rigid form, as in PVC pipes, making it one of the most adaptable and popular synthetics manufactured.

By the 1930s vinyl was promoted as a hygienic, durable, and fashionable alternative to traditional upholstery fabrics. Yet the slick surface qualities of the material proved unpopular to a public taken with the sensuous textures of woven materials. By mid-century, "breathable" vinyls for upholstery were advertised; these allowed air to pass through the material, keeping the vinyl "cool and dry," and lessening the friction of human skin on the manufactured surface. The Barbie doll, whose hard vinyl form withstands abuse from children, was introduced in 1959.

Vinyl simulacra of natural materials last longer and require less care than their natural counterparts. While it is an inexpensive alternative to the materials it sought to emulate, vinyl is also prized for its inherent qualities. By the 1960s, this dualism in the symbolic character of vinyl made itself apparent in the products available to consumers. At this time, vinyl floor tiles and wallcoverings were available in a large array of patterns. While some of these designs co-opted images and designs from popular culture, many tried to simulate the surface qualities of rarer materials such as marble, oak, and slate. The inflatable PVC furniture of the 1960s defied conventional forms in home decor, celebrating the man-made, the impermanent, and the inexpensive.

Contemporary vinyl objects reiterate this dichotomy between emulation and self-celebration. Vinyl fencing, siding, and flooring are often formed to imitate the look of natural materials, such as wood. Vinyl windows and flexible safety wrap used on food and medicines are modern membranes, dissolving notions of inside and out while still serving a protective function. Many vinyl products combine the qualities of traditional materials with vinyl's own attributes. A recently developed vinyl-flooring product bands together thin strips of the material so that it takes on the texture of a woven carpet while retaining vinyl's practical properties and synthetic sheen. R M

SKINDEX

Index compiled by Linda Lee

ADDITIONAL CREDITS: page 38, hand mixer: Collection of Cooper-Hewitt, National Design Museum, Smithsonian Institution, The Decorative Arts Association Acquisitions Fund, 1993-150-26-a. Photography: Matt Flynn.

Book design

ELLEN LUPTON

Editors

ELIZABETH JOHNSON
Cooper-Hewitt
National Design Museum
Smithsonian Institution
and

MARK LAMSTER
Princeton Architectural Press

Authors

ELLEN LUPTON is curator of contemporary design at Cooper-Hewitt, National Design Museum, Smithsonian Institution. She has organized many major exhibitions on twentieth- and twenty-first-century design at the museum, including *National Design Triennial: Design Culture Now* (2000); *Graphic Design in the Mechanical Age: Selections from the Merrill C. Berman Collection* (1999); *Mixing Messages: Graphic Design in Contemporary Culture* (1996); *The Avant-Garde Letterhead* (1996); and *Mechanical Brides: Women and Machines from Home to Office* (1993).

JENNIFER TOBIAS is Associate Librarian, Reference, Museum of Modern Art, New York City. She is pursuing her Ph.D. in Art History at the Graduate Center, City University of New York. She holds a Masters of Library Science from Rutgers University and a Bachelor of Fine Arts from The Cooper Union. Exhibitions organized at MoMA include *Modern Art and Reactionary Criticism* (Library, 2000) and "The Armory Show" in *Modern Starts: 1880–1920* (1999). She has written essays for *Library Trends* and other publications.

ALICIA IMPERIALE, artist and architect, is an Assistant Professor at Columbia University, Barnard College, and Pratt Institute in New York City, and at the Cornell University in Rome program. In 1998 she co-curated a traveling exhibit on young American architects called *architecture @ the edge*. She is the author of *New Flatness: Surface Tension in Digital Architecture* (2000). She has lectured internationally and is currently researching a book on the role of digital scanning technologies in the work of artists, architects, dancers, and theorists.

GRACE JEFFERS is a partner in the office of Inside Design, New York City, a firm dedicated to forward-thinking design development and education. She is also the curator of the Ralph and Sunny Wilson Historic House Museum in Temple, Texas, a house that pioneered the use of sheet plastics in interiors. Jeffers has received numerous awards, including the National Merit Award for Historic Preservation, the Metropolitan Home Modernism Award, and the Chicago Athenaeum Good Design Award. She is a graduate of The Art Institute of Chicago and The Bard Graduate Center for Studies in the Decorative Arts.

RANDI MATES is a masters candidate at the Bard Graduate Center for Studies in the Decorative Arts, Design, and Culture and a curatorial assistant at Cooper-Hewitt, National Design Museum. Her research focuses on the intersections of technology and material culture in the twentieth century, as well as twentieth-century graphic design and ephemera.

Typography

QUADRAAT
designed by FRED SMEIJERS, 1992
VAG ROUNDED
adapted from a nineteenth-century
grotesque for Volkswagen AG, 1979